The DSM-IV
Internet Companion

The DSM~IV
Internet Companion

M. Robert Morrison
Robert F. Stamps

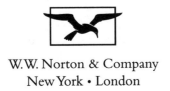

W.W. Norton & Company
New York • London

Printed in the United States of America
First Edition

Composition by Ken Gross
Manufacturing by Hamilton Printing
Book design by Ken Gross

Library of Congress Cataloging-in-Publication Data

Morrison, M. Robert, 1933–
  The DSM-IV internet companion / M. Robert Morrison,
Robert F. Stamps.
    p.   cm.
  "A Norton professional book"
  ISBN 0-393-70267-7 (pbk.)
  1. Psychiatry—Computer network resources. 2. Mental
health—Computer network resources. 3. Internet (Computer
network) I. Stamps, Robert F., 1950–   . II. Title.
RC437.2.M67 1998
025.06'61689—dc21   98-9971   CIP

W. W. Norton & Company, Inc., 500 Fifth Avenue, New York, N.Y. 10110
http://www.wwnorton.com
W. W. Norton & Company Ltd., 10 Coptic Street, London WC1A 1PU

3   4   5   6   7   8   9   0

In loving memory of
Joanne Morrison Franklin
and
Charlotte Stamps

Contents

Introduction

World Wide Web Sites

The bread and butter of the *DSM-IV Internet Companion* consists of individual web sites that are posted to the Internet by universities, companies, clinics, individuals, governments, and libraries. Although the web sites detailed in this book all relate to mental health in one way or another, the World Wide Web is a repository for information on virtually any topic under the sun (and often beyond it).

Web sites (or URL's) may be modified or removed from circulation at any time by their sponsors. It is not particularly difficult or expensive to maintain a web site; once most web sites are posted, they will remain in service for many years, particularly when their sponsors know their pages are useful to the people who access them.

It would not be unexpected, then, for a small percentage of the sites detailed in this book to be removed from circulation over a period of time. There are several dozen psychology search engines profiled in Chapter 2; use these "electronic directories" to find information on a particular topic should you find that any page listed is no longer in service or should you wish additional information on a topic you've already explored.

Chapter 1 lists approximately 1,000 URL's that relate directly to the diagnosis and treatment of the mental disorders found in the *DSM-IV*. These pages constitute a substantial body of knowledge and have great utility in and of themselves.

Remember, however, that new web sites (like new books in print) appear on a regular basis. The way to find them is to use the search engines listed in Chapter 2. These search engines are managed by professionals worldwide who are constantly monitoring the World Wide Web for fresh sites to add to their lists.

Chapter 1 is organized to follow the *DSM-IV* category by category. As mentioned, Chapter 2 is a compilation of psychology- and psychiatry-related directories. Chapters 3 and 4 list web sites that have relevance to some or to all of the *DSM-IV* disorders, and that is why they are not listed individually in Chapter 1.

Mailing Lists

Mailing lists allow subscribers to send e-mail messages to all other subscribers by simply submitting their message to the appropriate address. Mailing lists are built around individual topics, and contributors are expected to address that subject only. Mailing lists usually have between several dozen and several hundred members; a few lists have several thousand subscribers.

The vast majority of mailing lists are open, meaning that one can subscribe simply by contacting the list administrator and entering the appropriate subscription command. These commands differ slightly from list to list; the commands for the lists detailed below are supplied. The mailing lists described in each chapter generally have open subscription.

Closed lists have more discriminating admission policies. Many closed lists are open only to qualified professionals with particular interest in the subject at hand. A subscriber who attempts to subscribe to a closed list will be given instructions for admission.

List subscribers may expect to receive as few as a handful of messages per month and as many as several dozen per day. It's difficult to gauge the amount of messages generated in any individual list; it is important, therefore, that subscribers be prepared to remove themselves should they find the amount of messages excessive or their quality insufficient. Unsubscribing is a simple procedure as long as one knows the correct command. List administrators will frequently list all relevant commands as a postscript to many messages. In America, the words "subscribe" or "unsubscribe" are typically used; in the United Kingdom the commands used are frequently "join" and "leave."

A mailing list can be a very valuable source of information and personal contact. It can unite interested parties from around the world in stimulating discussion and debate. It can also, unfortunately, become a source of constant irritation. Some mailing lists are little more than "chat rooms" where people with nothing better to do communicate casually with other people in the same situation. And stimulating debate sometimes degenerates into offensive personal attacks.

Approach mailing lists with cautious optimism. They do, on occasion, provide priceless advice and counsel. Make sure, however, that unsubscribing can be done should the need arise.

Mailing lists are supplied at the end of each section where they have relevance.

Usenet Groups

Usenet or news groups are similar to mailing lists, but news group messages must be accessed manually. No one "belongs" to a news group; messages are instead posted to an electronic bulletin board that can be accessed through the computer user's browser and local Internet service provider. Messages remain on line from a few days to a few weeks. Interested parties may read messages or post them for others to read.

Individual news groups are not listed in this book; they are very easy to find, and many of them come and go in just a few months.

Deja News <http://www.dejanews.com> is the World Wide Web's best way to find news groups. A recent search of "psychology" yielded a total of 9,225 lists with some relevance to the subject. Many psychology- and psychiatry-related search engines listed in Chapter 2 will also supply addresses for certain groups. News groups are available in virtually every topic imaginable.

Finding News Groups <http://www.ii.com/internet/messaging/newsgroups/> from Infinite Ink is another good way to locate them, and it has instructions on how to use them properly as well.

Web Sites with DSM or ICD Codes

DSM-IV Codes

The following sites provide code numbers only; they are not a substitute for the *DSM-IV*. The *DSM-IV* is published by the American Psychiatric Press and can be ordered by calling (800) 368-5777.

1. <http://uhs.bsd.uchicago.edu/dr-bob/tips/unframed/dsm4n.html>
    DSM-IV Diagnoses and Codes, Numerical Listing
    > From Dr. Bob's Virtual Encyclopedia.

2. <http://www.vghtpe.gov.tw/~psy/cclin/dsm4a.htm>
    Alphabetical Listing of DSM-IV Diagnoses and Codes
    > An easy to use site from the Veteran's General Hospital in Taipei, Taiwan.

3. <http://psy.utmb.edu/disorder/dsm4/dsmnum.htm>
    DSM-IV Diagnoses and Codes—Numerical List
    > From the University of Texas Medical Branch at Galveston.

ICD Codes

4. <http://www.informatik.fh-luebeck.de/icd/List.html>
    List of ICD-10 Categories for Mental Disorders
    - From Technische Informatik at the University of Lubeck in Germany.
    - Codes are in English.

Chapter 1
The *DSM~IV* Disorders

SECTION I.
Disorders Usually First Diagnosed in Infancy, Childhood, or Adolescence

The *DSM-IV* includes the following disorders:

A. Mental Retardation, characterized by significantly subaverage intellectual functioning.

B. Learning Disorders, characterized by academic functioning below chronological age, measured intelligence, and age-appropriate education.

C. Motor Skills Disorders, characterized by motor coordination substantially below expected chronological age and measured intelligence.

D. Communication Disorders, characterized by difficulties in speech or language.

E. Pervasive Developmental Disorders, characterized by severe deficits, and pervasive impairment in multiple areas of development.

F. Attention-Deficit and Disruptive Behavior Disorders, characterized by prominent symptoms of inattention and/or hyperactivity-impulsivity.

G. Feeding and Eating Disorders of Infancy or Early Childhood, characterized by persistent disturbances in feeding and eating.

H. Tic Disorders, characterized by vocal and/or motor tics.

I. Elimination Disorders, usually divided into Encopresis and Enuresis.

    J. Other Disorders:
        i.   Separation Anxiety
        ii. Selective Mutism
        iii. Reactive Attachment Disorders
        iv. Stereotypic Movement Disorders
    K. Others
        i.   Down Syndrome. Although not included as a distinct category in the *DSM-IV,* Down Syndrome is a major disorder in pre-natal development and manifests many of the disorders contained in the section dealing with disorders first diagnosed in infancy, childhood or adolescence. Important additional information in working with children
        ii. Special Needs

A. *Mental Retardation*

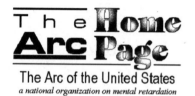

http://TheArc.org/welcome.html
The Arc Home Page ★
Arlington, Texas

> The largest voluntary organization dedicated to mental retardation. National headquarters is located in Arlington, Texas. Arc has over a thousand affiliated chapters. Contains many divisions, including a Department of Research and Program Services.

http://www.circ.uab.edu/
Civitan International Research Center ★
University of Alabama, Birmingham, Alabama

> Research Center at University of Alabama, Birmingham, devoted to improving well-being and quality of life of individuals and families affected by mental retardation and developmental disabilities. Many hyperlinks.

http://www.familyvillage.wisc.edu/
Family Village ★

> Sponsored in part by Joseph P. Kennedy Foundation and Mitsubishi Electric America Foundation, Family Village is a global community that integrates information, resources, and communication opportunities on the Internet for persons with mental retardation and other disabilities, their families, and others providing services and support. Extensive and contains many hyperlinks.

http://www.FRAXA.org/
Fragile X Syndrome Research Foundation ★

This syndrome is the #1 inherited cause of mental retardation. Article describes symptoms, cause, new diagnostic tests and treatment. The Research Foundation is a non-profit organization run by parents and medical professionals made up entirely of volunteers.

http://TheArc.org/faqs/group.html
Group Counseling for People with Mental Retardation

The use of group counseling for people with mental retardation and developmental disabilities has traditionally been limited. Authors claim that this is a treatment whose time has come and recommends its use for issues dealing with anger management, AIDS awareness, relationship and sexual issues. Article explains the advantages of group therapy; the Interactive and Behavioral model; issues Related to Group Therapy; Conclusions.

http://teach.virginia.edu/go/cise/ose/categories/mr.html
Mental Retardation ★

Excellent hyperlinks to general issues dealing with Mental Retardation; Organizations for the Mentally Retarded; General Resources on Mental Retardation; Down Syndrome Resources; Special Olympics Information; Mental Retardation Centers and Departments.

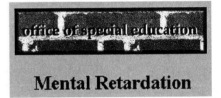

Mental Retardation

http://www.psych-health.com/link-mr.htm
Mental Retardation Links ★

Hyperlinks to Associations for Mental Retardation and Other Developmental Disabilities. From the California Association of Psychiatric Technicians.

http://busboy.sped.ukans.edu/~music/resources/mr/mr.shtml
Mental Retardation Resources ★

Hyperlinks to various resources and organizations dealing with Mental Retardation.

B. *Learning Disorders*

i. DYSLEXIA

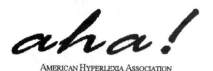

AMERICAN HYPERLEXIA ASSOCIATION

http://www.hyperlexia.org/
American Hyperlexic Association Home Page ★
Elmhurst, Illinois
AHA is a non-profit organization comprised of people interested in the syndrome called Hyperlexia, which has characteristics similar to autism, behavior disorder, language disorder, emotional disorder, ADD, hearing impairment, giftedness or mental retardation. Hyperlexia is a syndrome observed in children with the following characteristics: precocious ability to read words above what would be expected; significant difficulty in understanding verbal language; abnormal social skills with difficulty in socializing and interacting appropriately with people.

http://www.hensa.ac.uk/dyslexia.html
Dyslexia Archives ★
U.K.
Funded by Higher Education Funding Council for England, DA is a collection of up-to-date materials covering all aspects of dyslexia. Specifically designed to make it easy for anyone to find, read, and retrieve information needed to understand dyslexia.

http://www.sofdesign.com/dyslexia/
Dyslexia Training Program
From the Texas Scottish Rite Hospital for Children, offers videotape instructional and computer-based programs.

http://www.monash.edu.au/informatics/idcn.html
Intellectual Disability Network ★★
Extensive hyperlinks to all issues dealing with intellectual disabilities. A must for professionals and researchers! From Monash University, Victoria, Australia.

http://www.interdys.org/about_od.stm
International Dyslexia Association ★
Baltimore, Maryland
International non-profit association dedicated to the study and treatment of dyslexia. Established to continue pioneering work of Dr. Orton, one of the first to study this disorder. Contains hyperlinks to variety of resources including research, legal and legislative issues.

http://www.ldanatl.org/
Learning Disabilities Association ★
Pittsburgh, Pennsylvania

> National non-profit organization to advance education and general welfare of children and adults of normal or potentially normal intelligence who manifest handicaps of a perceptual, conceptual, or coordinative nature. Valuable hyperlinks.

Learning Disabilities Association

Welcome! The Learning Disabilities Association of America is a national, non-profit organization. Our purpose is to advance the education and general welfare of children and adults of normal or potentially normal intelligence who manifest handicaps of a perceptual, conceptual, or coordinative nature.

http://www.rfbd.org/
Recording for the Blind and Dyxlexic ★
Princeton, New Jersey

Providing service for a half century, RFB&D is a national non-profit organization that serves people who cannot read standard print because of a visual, perceptual, or physical disability. The leading library of academic and professional textbooks on audiotape from elementary through postgraduate level.

http://www.schoolnet.ca/sne/
Special Needs Education Network

> A Canadian-sponsored site which provides Internet resources for parents, teachers, and other professionals involved in the education of students with special needs.

http://www.vsarts.org/
Very Special Arts

> Non-profit organization with a mission to promote arts, education and creative expression involving children and adults with disabilities. Hyperlinks to a variety of resources.

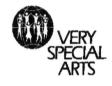

ii. OTHER

http://adhostnt.adhost.com/cgi-win/athealth32.exe?39
Mathematics Disorder

> Describes the disorder, genetic factors, age at onset, etc.

http://adhostnt.adhost/com/cgi-win/athealth32.exe?38
Reading Disorder

> Describes reading disorder, genetic factors, age of onset, diagnosis, etc.

http://adhostnt.adhost/com/cgi-win/athleath32.exe?40
Written Expression Disorder

> Describes written expression disorder, signs of the disorder, gender, age at onset, etc.

C. *Motor Skills Disorders*

No articles solely related to this disorder appear on the Internet. This disorder is often included in articles dealing with general disorders in this category.

D. *Communication Disorders*

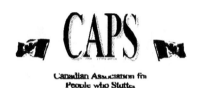

Canadian Association for People who Stutter

http://www.webcon.net/~caps/intro.html
Canadian Association for People Who Stutter
Canada
> Since 1995, Association has provided people who stutter, their family and friends, speech-language pathologists, academics, students and the general public with information on stuttering resources available both in and outside Canada.

http://ecuvax.cis.ecu/academics/schdept/ah/csd/Stutt.html
East Carolina University's Stuttering Page ★
> Contains hyperlinks to listing of researchers in speech disorders at ECU; a videotape for clinicians and researchers; conference abstracts; summary of studies.

http://www.xs4all.nl/~edorlow/isa.html
International Stuttering Association ★
> Listing of ISA projects and links to member organizations from countries all over the world.

http://www.stuttering.com/
National Center for Stuttering ★
New York, New York
> Established in 1976. Provides up-to-date information about stuttering. Links to National Stutterer's Hotline. Cites research regarding causes and treatments. Member associations in many countries.

Welcome to the Home Page of
The National Center For Stuttering

http://members.aol.com/nsphome/index.html
National Stuttering Project Home Page
Anaheim Hills, California
> The NSP was founded in 1977 to let stutterers know and experience the fact that they are not alone in facing this challenge. The NSP serves as an advocate for stutterers and raises the consciousness of the general public about this disorder through education and outreach activities.

THE SPEECH-LANGUAGE PATHOLOGY
WEBSITE

http://www.ica.net/pages/fred/
Speech-Language Pathology Website ★
> Provides information to anyone interested in learning about speech and language development and associated disorders. Discusses normal speech and language development, speech-sound development, disorder vs. delay, etc. Links to other sites dealing with related topics.

http://www.mankato.msus.edu/dept/comdis/kuster/Kehoe/
ADA.html

Stuttering, Employment and the Americans With Disabilities Act

Discusses a case of discrimination based on stuttering; the American With Disabilities Act; myths about people who stutter; principle of reasonable accommodation; free money from the IRS for stutterers; whom to contact; how to handle interviews.

http://www.mankato.msus.edu/dept/comdis/kuster/stutter.html

Stuttering Homepage ★★

Dedicated to providing information about stuttering. Contains many hyperlinks to information; discussion forums; conference information; non-English information; stuttering course syllabi; research; therapy; etc. Also contains links to a page Just for Kids and Just for Teens.

The Stuttering Homepage

Information about Stuttering	Discussion forums about stuttering	PWS speak for themselves	Conference Information
Non-English Information about Stuttering	Stuttering in the popular media	Creative Expression	Stuttering Course Syllabi
Cluttering and other related fluency disorders	Public Relations - Spreading the Word	People who don't stutter share information	Research on Stuttering
Therapy for Stuttering	Hall of Fame and The Pioneers	On the Lighter Side	Some information about communication
Support Organizations for PWS	The Bookstore	Personal Paths Toward Recovery & Case Studies	Other homepages about stuttering
NEW What's New	Just for Kids	Just for Teens	"Hello World," Charles Van Riper

Stuttering Home Page Chat Room - sponsored by Key City Sertoma

http://www.casafuturatech.com

Stuttering: Science, Therapy and Practice ★

An online book with excellent hyperlinks to science, therapy, and practice. Practical resources.

http://www.prevent_stuttering.com

Stuttering Prevention ★

Dedicated to providing information about the nature of stuttering and ways to prevent its development. Contains articles about early childhood stuttering, including warning signs, ways to reduce communication demands for children and intervention programs for preventing and treating early childhood stuttering. Many hyperlinks to other articles about stuttering in school-aged children and adults.

http://www.mankato.msus.edu/dept/comdis/kuster/
TherapyWWW/srf/states.html

Therapy Programs by State

The Stuttering Resource Project presents a directory of programs that provide services in the U.S. to people who stutter. Hyperlinks to most states as well as Canadian and international organizations.

http://members.aol.com/wdparry/valsalva.htm

Valsalva Mechanism

Shows how a natural bodily function, Valsalva mechanism, may turn efforts to speak into the blocks we are trying to avoid. Explains how a combination of physical and psychological factors may trap us in a Valsalva-stuttering cycle, which may actually trigger and perpetuate stuttering.

E. *Pervasive Developmental Disorders*

i. AUTISM

http://www.latitudes.org/
Association for Comprehensive NeuroTherapy
Royal Palm Beach, Florida
> Explores advanced and alternative treatment for neurological conditions. ACN is a forum through which practitioners and laypersons can communicate about diverse, non-drug approaches to neurological conditions. Attempts to provide latest information in the field while promoting related studies and research.

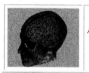

http://nodulus.extern.ucsd.edu/
Autism and Brain Development Research Laboratory
San Diego, California
> In conjunction with Children's Hospital, San Diego and UCSD, discusses neurophysiological and neuroanatomical basis of autism. Studies the cerebellar and cerebral anatomical abnormalities as well the attentional difficulties common to autism with the use of MRI's, functional MRI's, event-related brain potentials, and reaction time behavioral tests.

http://WWW.FRS-INC.COM/
Autism and Developmental Delay Resource Catalog
> Catalog which includes books on autism, developmental disabilities, ADD/ADHD. Developed by parents of an autistic child.

http://www.onramp.net/autism/conf1.html
Autism Conferences
> Listing all autism conferences in the U.S. Wonderful resource for professionals.

http://www.ability.org.uk/autism.html
Autism Index ★
> Contains hyperlinks dealing with all aspects of autism. Contains an Index Page, A–Z Index, Search Engine, Other Links. Invaluable for persons interested in this disorder. From Ability in Gloucestershire, U.K.

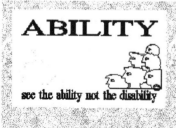

http://www.autism.com/ari/
Autism Research Institute: Research
San Diego, California
> The Autism Research Institute offers references to research on autism.

http://web.syr.edu/~jmwobus/autism/
Autism Resources ★
   Index of online information and resources on the developmental disabilities of autism and Asperger's. An organized list of resources about autism, with links for any site dealing with Autism. Invaluable resource.

http://www.autism-society.org/
Autism Society of America ★
Bethesda, Maryland
   Serving the needs of individuals with autism and their families through advocacy, education, public awareness, and research since 1965, ASA offers information regarding the nature of autism, advice, education, conferences, as well as a glossary of terms and abbreviations.

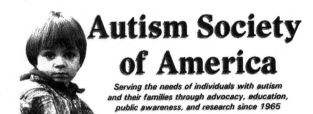

Autism Society of America

Serving the needs of individuals with autism and their families through advocacy, education, public awareness, and research since 1965

http://www.mentalhealth.com/dis1/p21-ch06.html
Autistic Disorder: American Description
   Presents criteria for diagnosis of Autistic Disorder.

http://www.injersey.com/Living/Health/Autism/page3.html
Diagnosing Autism and Other Pervasive Developmental Disorders
   Thomas Boyle presents extensive information about diagnosing autism.

http://www.geocities.com/HotSprings/8442/whiteind.htm
Jypsy's Autism, AS, MS, Homepage ★
   Personal story with excellent resources for booklets, other hyperlinks, autism in other languages, links to other search engines, etc.

http://www.autism.org/pdd.html
Plain Talk about PDD and the Diagnosis of Autism
   By Bernard Rimland. PDD is discussed as a poorly understood, uninformative, confusing, and unpopular label which should be abandoned. Claims that PDD is a label concocted by psychiatrists to cover up the fact that they are uncertain about a particular disorder.

ii. RETT'S DISORDER

http://www2.paltech.com/irsa/irsa.htm
International Rett Syndrome Association
Clinton, Maryland
   The mission of the IRSA is to support and encourage medical research to determine the cause and find a cure for Rett syndrome, to increase public awareness of Rett syndrome, and to provide informational and emotional support to families of children with Rett syndrome.

INTERNATIONAL RETT SYNDROME ASSOCIATION

WELCOME TO IRSA

The mission of the IRSA is to support and encourage medical reseach to determine the cause and find a cure for Rett syndrome, to increase public awareness of Rett syndrome, and to provide informational and emotional support to families of children with Rett syndrome.

iii. CHILDHOOD DISINTEGRATIVE DISORDER

No articles specific to this disorder appear on the Internet. However, this may be covered in general Internet articles dealing with other disorders in this section.

iv. ASPERGER'S SYNDROME

http//amug.org/~a203/table_contents.html
Asperger/Autism: On-The-Same-Page
> Articles and information about international projects and autism in various countries. Discusses international rights of the disabled: English, French, Spanish.

http://www.rmplc.co.uk/eduweb/sites/autism/autism7.html# main
Autism—High Functioning, Asperger's Syndrome ★
Kettering, Northants, UK
> From the Society For The Autistically Handicapped, presents diagnostic information and common features. Also contains worldwide hyperlinks.

http://www.ummed.edu/pub/o/ozbayrak/asperger.html
Asperger's Disorder Homepage ★
> Describes the epidemiology of Asperger's; differences between Asperger's and high-functioning autism; biology of Asperger's; diagnostic criteria; treatment; and a listing of clinicians from the U.S. and other countries who evaluate Asperger's.

http://www.autism.org/asperger.html
Asperger's Syndrome
> Lists behaviors of individuals with Asperger's Syndrome.

http://www.wpi.edu/%7Etrek/aspergers.html
Asperger's Syndrome
> Definitions of Asperger's and important hyperlinks to other Resources. From Amy Marr.

http://www.autism.org/asperger.html
Asperger's Syndrome
> Lists behaviors of individuals with Asperger's Syndrome.

On-Line Asperger Syndrome Information and Support
(A.K.A. Asperger Syndrome Resources)

http://www.udel.edu/bkirby/asperger/
Asperger Syndrome: OASIS ★★
> The most comprehensive source for hyperlinks to: research papers and description of AS; description of related disorders; current research projects; educational implications; computers and software; social implications; legal information; listing of universities, medical centers and clinicians who evaluate for AS.

http://www.vicnet.net.au/vicnet/community/asperger.htm
Asperger's Syndrome Support Network Homepage
Victoria Australia

> Describes all aspects of Asperger's Syndrome children. Intends to help Australians and New Zealanders cope with feelings of being alone in the situation, providing a sense of community, identifying local resources and being able to share and discuss information and lifestyle issues. Assisting at the grassroots level.

http://www.gifu-kyoiku.ac.jp:10070/home/tsujii/eng/aspinv.
html
Invitation for Asperger Society ★
Japan

> Formed in 1992, AD is a organization for and about people with high-functioning pervasive developmental disorder (PDD), including Asperger Syndrome. AS has three special interest groups: (1) Children's and Parents' Group, (2) Asperger Society Supporters Club, (3) Asperger Society Friendly Club.

F. *Attention~Deficit and Disruptive Behavior Disorders*

i. ATTENTION~DEFICIT DISORDER

http://www.register.com/family-matters/p0000708.htm
ADD/ADHD Information Library ★

> Information for parents on ADD/ADHD, including diagnosis, treatment options, resources for families. Contains hyperlinks to Dr. Cowan's ADD lectures.

http://www.nlci.com/nutrition/
ADD/ADHD Online Newsletter

> A publication for helping children and adults with ADHD. Emphasis is on nutrition.

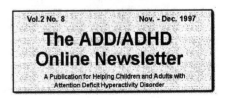

Vol. 2 No. 8   Nov. - Dec. 1997
The ADD/ADHD Online Newsletter
A Publication for Helping Children and Adults with Attention Deficit Hyperactivity Disorder

http://www3.sympatico.ca/frankk/contents.html
ADD: FAQ

> FAQ broken into 6 sections: background; treatments; sources of information; miscellaneous information; recent updates; adult ADD tests.

http://www.signasoft.com/addult
ADDult Recovery ★

> A twelve-step program for ADD. Hyperlinks to information regarding ADD Conferences and Meetings, sites on the Internet, ADDulthood Newsletter, resources. From Angie Dixon.

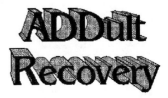

http://www.mentalhealth.com/dis1/p21-ch01.html
American Description: Diagnostic Criteria
Diagnostic criteria for ADHD.

http://www.apa.org/books/adhabs.html
ADHD: Abstracts of Psychological and Behavioral Literature
An annotated bibliography of journal abstracts, dissertations and books written about this disorder from 1971 to 1994.

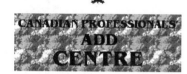

http://www.usask.ca/psychiatry/CPADDC.html
Canadian Professionals ADD Page ★
Designed for Canadian teachers, counselors, psychologists, nurses, physicians, neurologists, and anyone with a professional interest in assisting people with ADHD and their families. Offers information, services, meetings, etc.

http://www.chadd.org/
CH.A.D.D. ★
Plantation, Florida
A non-profit parent-based organization formed to better the lives of individuals with ADD. Through family support and advocacy, public and professional education and encouragement of scientific research, CH.A.D.D. works to insure that ADD people are given opportunities to reach their inherent potential.

http://www.eegspectrum.com
EEG Spectrum
Encino, California
Research and training center for treating ADD/ADHD and other disorders through EEG biofeedback.

http://www.feingold.org/
Feingold Association Dietary Connection
Dietary connections to better behavior, learning and health. Contains index from A to Z.

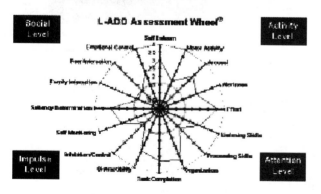

http://www.addmed.com/addmed/add/pages/diagnos.htm
L-ADD Assessment Wheel
Canadian Anthony Laws developed a comprehensive diagnostic assessment and treatment tool used to assist in the clinical diagnosis of ADD in children, adolescents, and adults. Instrument contains 16 booklets designed to be age and location specific.

http://www.addmtc.com/tenneur.html
Neurological Behaviors Characteristic of ADD
> Ten neurological behaviors characteristic of ADD/ADHD. From the ADD Medical Treatment Center of Santa Clara Valley, California

http://www.mindspring.com/~staywell/add.html
Nutritional Supplement for ADD
> Reviews common symptoms of ADD and nutritional alternative to drugs.

http://www.mentalhealth.com/dis-rs3/p26-ch01.html
Research regarding Cause of ADHD ★
> Comprehensive summary of research studies regarding the cause of ADHD.

http://www.mentalhealth.com/dis-rs/p24-ch01.html
Research regarding Diagnosis of ADHD ★
> Comprehensive summary of research studies regarding the diagnosis of ADHD.

http://www.mentalhealth.com/dis-rs2/p25-ch01.html
Research regarding Treatment ★
> Comprehensive summary of research studies regarding the treatment of ADHD.

ii. DISRUPTIVE BEHAVIOR DISORDERS

http://www.nlbbs.com/~jstewart/
Understanding and Managing the Aggressive and Acting-Out Child in the Public School Setting
> Video series designed to provide training to teachers, counselors, administrators and psychologists who work with behaviorally handicapped/emotionally disturbed children within a public school setting.

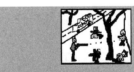

Understanding and Managing the Aggressive and Acting-Out Child in the Public School Setting

http://www.mentalhealth.com/dis1/p21-ch02.html
Conduct Disorder: American Description
> Diagnostic criteria for Conduct Disorder.

http://www.mentalhealth.org/CHILD/CONDUCT.HTM
Conduct Disorder in Children and Adolescents Fact Sheet
> From Center for Mental Health Services, refers to the range of all diagnosable emotional, behavioral, and mental disorders. These include depression, ADD, ADHD, anxiety, conduct and eating disorders.

http://www.mentalhealth.com/dis-rs1/p24-ch02.html
Conduct Disorder: Research regarding Diagnosis ★
> Comprehensive summary of research studies dealing with diagnosis of Conduct Disorder.

Conduct Disorder

Research Re: Treatment

http://www.mentalhealth.com/dis-rs2/p25-ch02.html
Conduct Disorder: Research regarding Treatment ★
> Comprehensive summary of research studies dealing with treatment of Conduct Disorder.

http://www.mentalhealth.com/dis1/p21-ch05.html
Oppositional Defiant Disorder: American Description
> Diagnostic criteria, associated features and differential diagnosis of Oppositional Defiant Disorder.

http://www.mentalhealth.com/dis-rs1/p24-ch05.html
Oppositional Defiant Disorder: Research regarding Diagnosis ★
> Comprehensive summary of research regarding diagnosis of Oppositional Defiant Disorder.

http://www.mentalhealth.com/rx/p23-ch05.html
Oppositional Defiant Disorder: Treatment
> Presents medical and psychosocial treatments for Oppositional Defiant Disorder.

G. *Feeding and Eating Disorders*

http://www.cmhc.com/disorders/sx74.htm
Pica: Symptoms
> Very brief explanation of Pica symptoms.

http://www.cmhc.com/disorders/sx77.htm
Rumination Disorder
> Very brief explanation of Rumination disorder.

H. *Tic Disorders*

DAILY PARENT
Tourette's Syndrome

http://www.dailyparent.com/dailyp/source/article/1257.html
Daily Parent: Helping Children Who Have Tourette's
> Live chat room; discussion and forums. Hyperlinks to parenting, education, health, family, children, food, money, living arts, home, careers, your world.

http://neuro-www2.mgh.harvard.edu/TSA/medsci/definitions.html
Definitions and Classification of Tic Disorders
> Defines and classifies the various tic disorders

http://www.mentalhealth.com/book/p40-gtor.html
Guide to the Diagnosis and Treatment of Tourette Syndrome ★
> Comprehensive article dealing with Tourette Syndrome and other tic disorders; clinical assessment of Tourette Syndrome; treatment of Tourette Syndrome; references.

http://www.mentalhealth.com/dis1/p21-ch04.html
Tourette's Disorder: American Description
> Diagnostic criteria, associated features and differential diagnosis for Tourette's.

http://www-personal.umd.umich.edu/~infinit/ts-contents.html
Tourette Syndrome: Frequently Asked Questions
> Discusses what Tourette Syndrome is, living with Tourette Syndrome, what next? Good hyperlinks.

http://www.cmhc.com/disorders/sx82.htm
Transient Tic Disorder: Symptoms
> Brief description of symptoms of Transient Tic Disorder.

http://www.vh.org/Patients/IHB/Psych/Tourette/HomePage
.html
Virtual Hospital: Tourette Syndrome
University of Iowa
> From University of Iowa Department of Psychiatry and Tourette Syndrome Association. Contains hyperlinks to definitions; medical information; academic/school information; patient/family information; and other Internet sites.

I. *Elimination Disorders*

http://kidshealth.org/parent/healthy/enuresis.html
Bedwetting: What Parents Need to Know
> Discusses facts parents need to know; who's affected; what can be done; kinds of enuresis; potential for a cure; successful treatments.

http://village.ios.com/~tis/child.html
Childhood Incontinence ★
> Excellent description of Childhood Incontinence from Tri-state Incontinence Support Group.

http://avery.med.virginia.edu/~smb4v/tutorials/constipation/
constip.htm
Chronic Constipation ★
> Discusses chronic constipation with many hyperlinks to why does it happen and symptoms and treatments. Also hyperlinks to articles explaining encopresis.

http://www.rxmed.com/illnesses/encopresis.html
Encopresis
> Quick medical overview looking at causes; signs and symptoms; risk factors; prevention; diagnosis and treatment; medications; activity; diet; possible complications; prognosis.

http://www.nafc.org/whatis_frame.html
National Association for Continence ★
Spartanburg, South Carolina

> Founded in 1982 NACF is a non-profit organization dedicated to improving quality of life of people with incontinence. NAFC's purpose is to be the leading source of education, advocacy and support to the public and the health professional about the causes, prevention, diagnosis, treatments, and management alternatives for incontinence.

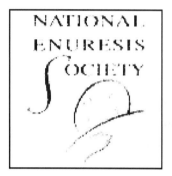

http://www.peds.umn.edu/Centers/NES/
National Enuresis Society ★
Dallas, Texas

> A non-profit organization of doctors and others building greater awareness and understanding of enuresis. Excellent resources with many hyperlinks.

http://kidshealth.org/parent/healthy/enuresis.html
Wet Set: What Parents Need to Know About Bedwetting ★

> Great article for parents. Discusses who's affected; what can be done; kinds of enuresis; no answers, but a cure; successful treatments.

J. *Other Disorders*

i. SEPARATION ANXIETY

http://www.mentalhealth.com/dis1/p21-ch03.html
Separation Anxiety Disorder: American Description

> Diagnostic criteria, associated features, differential diagnosis.

ii. SELECTIVE MUTISM

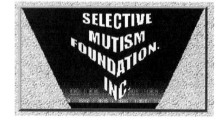

http://personal.mia.bellsouth.net/mia/g/a/garden/garden/
Selective Mutism Foundation

> A non-profit public service organization which offers information and promotes research about selective mutism.

http://www/flinet.com/~diverse/smg/index.html
Selective Mutism Group Web Site

> Dedicated to furthering research and offering support for selective mutism. Provided as a public service by a concerned parent who feels that all information should be made available to all people free of charge.

iii. REACTIVE ATTACHMENT DISORDER

http://www.attach-bond.com/
Attachment Home Page
> Dedicated to helping parents and children develop strong attachments and bonds as a way to security, self-esteem, and peace.

Keywords: attachment, attachment disorder, adoption, adopt, adopted, therapy, psychotherapy, bonding, bond, family, families, children, child, parenting, parents, mental health.

Attachment Home Page

This web site is dedicated to helping parents and children develop strong attachments and bonds. This, we believe, is the way to security, self-esteem, and peace. In our view, as a child, it is not possible to develop true self-esteem and find peace without resolving differences and emotional pain due to stressed or damaged emotional ties to your parents and family. At this site, you can find information and support in your endeavor to improve or heal your family.

http://www.sni.net/pwp
Attachment Disorders: Information and Effective Treatments ★
> Deborah Hage indicates that there is hope for children who have come through foster care and into adoption emotionally scared from abuse and neglect. Hyperlinks to further information, including therapy and consultation.

iv. STEREOTYPIC MOVEMENT DISORDER

http://www.movementdisorders.com
Movement Disorder Society
Woodbury, New Jersey
> Provides international forums to disseminate information on recent advances in movement disorders; enhances the education of physicians and public about movement disorders; offers information about the quality of care of patients with movement disorders through support of research and education.

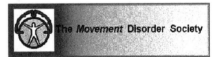

K. *Others*

i. DOWN SYNDROME

http://www.cmhc.com/factsfam/downsyn.htm
Down Syndrome ★
> Presents current information about Down syndrome for families and children with the disorder and those who care for them. Covers general information on all aspects of Down Syndrome. Many hyperlinks.

http://www.nas.com/downsyn/
Down Syndrome WWW Page ★
Established in 1995, the Down Syndrome WWW Page offers contemporary articles; FAQ; worldwide information and organizations; inclusion and education resources; parent matching and support groups; conferences.

▶ **Down Syndrome WWW Page**

ii. SPECIAL NEEDS

http://www.quasar.ualberta.ca/ddc/incl/intro.htm
Inclusion: School as a Caring Community
Offers support and resources to elementary and secondary teachers. Includes chapters on learning strategies, student evaluations, and teaching social needs.

http://www.schoolnet.ca/sne/
Special Needs Education Network
Sponsored by the Canadian government in conjunction with educators, this site provides Internet services to parents, teachers, schools, and other professionals and organization involved in the education of students with special needs.

http://www.specialolympics.org/
Special Olympics International ★
A program begun in 1968 by Eunice Kennedy Shriver, Special Olympics is an international program of year-round training and athletic competition for children and adults with mental retardation. In all 50 U.S. States and in 141 countries worldwide.

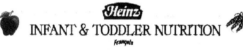

L. *Miscellaneous Sites of Interest*

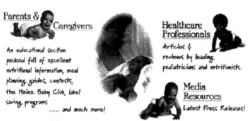

http://www.heinzbaby.com
Infant and Toddler Nutrition ★
Good information from the Heinz Corporation.

http://www.minorcon.org
A Minor Consideration
Paul Petersen's program to help child actors in trouble.

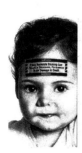

http://www.dss.cahwnet.gov/baby/default.htm
Shaken Baby Campaign
California Department of Social Services. Good basic information.

http://webster.state.nh.us/dhhs/ohm/iasbs.htm
Shaken Baby Syndrome
New Hampshire Department of Health and Human Services. A fact sheet for professionals.

http://www.williams-syndrome.org/
Williams Syndrome Association ★
Clawson, Michigan
> With 10 regions across America, WSA reaches out to
> assist individuals with Williams Syndrome.

http://www.wsf.org/wsf.htm
The Williams Syndrome Foundation
University of California, Irvine
> Funds medical and educational projects.

http://www.sos.on.ca/~pmackay/williams.html
Canadian Association for Williams Syndrome
Vancouver, British Colombia
> Good basic information.

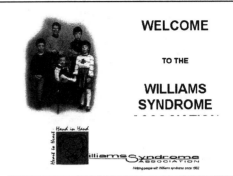

WELCOME
TO THE
WILLIAMS
SYNDROME

M. *Mailing Lists*

ADDKIDS: for Children with Attention
    Deficit Disorder
listserv@maelstrom.stjohns.edu
SUBSCRIBE ADDKIDS

ADD-MATE: for Spouses and Significant
    Others of Adults with ADD/ADHD
listserv@maelstrom.stjohns.edu
SUBSCRIBE ADD-MATE

ADDPARENTS: Support and Information
    Sharing for Parents with ADD children
listserver@bdtp.com
SUBSCRIBE ADDPARENTS

Twelve-Step Discussion for ADD
listserv@listserv.aol.com
SUBSCRIBE ADDULTANON

Autism
listserv@sjuvm.stjohns.edu
SUBSCRIBE AUTISM

Autinet Forum: Especially for High-Function
    Autism and Asperger's Syndrome
autinet-request@iol.ie
Place **subscribe** in the subject line. Explain
    your reasons for wanting to subscribe in
    the body of the message.

Autism Network International
listserv@listserv.syr.edu
SUBSCRIBE ANI-L

Behavior and Emotional Disorders in Children
listserv@asuvm.inre.asu.edu
sub BEHAVIOR Your Name

Children with Special Health Care Needs
listserv@lists.ufl.edu
sub CSHCN-L Your Name

Child Psychology
listserv@maelstrom.stjohns.edu
sub CAPSYCH Your Name

Children's Special Needs
listserv@netvm.nerdc.ufl.edu
SUBSCRIBE CSHCN-L Your Name

Communication Disorder Discussion
listserv@listserv.kent.edu
SUBSCRIBE CDMAJOR

Developmental Delays
majordomo@tbag.osc.edu
SUBSCRIBE OUR-KIDS

Developmental Disabilities
listserv@listserv.nodak.edu
SUBSCRIBE PSYCH-DD

Down Syndrome Discussion
listserv@ vm1.nodak.edu
DOWN-SYN Your Name

Down Syndrome Research
mailbase@mailbase.ac.uk
JOIN DOWNS-RESEARCH Your Name

Dyslexia
mailbase@mailbase.ac.uk
JOIN DYSLEXIA Your Name

Enuresis Support and Information Group
    (ESIG)
listserv@maelstrom.stjohns.edu
SUBSCRIBE ENURESIS

Incontinence
listserv@maine.maine.edu
SUBSCRIBE INCONT-L Your Name

Ingestive Behavior
listserv@cuvmb.bitnet
SUBSCRIBE INGEST

Learning Disabilities and Women
listserv@uga.cc.uga.edu
SUBSCRIBE LD-WOMEN Your Name

Mental Health Issues Related to Children and
    Teens
KMH-List-Request@affinitybooks.com
Ask to be included

Stuttering Research and Support
listserv@vm.temple.edu
SUB STUTT-L Your Name

Talented and Gifted Children's Discussion
    List
listserv@maelstrom.stjohns.edu
SUBSCRIBE TAGKIDS

Talented and Gifted Education
listserv@listserv.nodak.edu
SUBSCRIBE TAG-L

Tourette's Syndrome
majordomo@chebucto.ns.ca
SUBSCRIBE TOURETTE

No boundaries Tourette discussion
majordomo@chebucto.ns.ca
SUBSCRIBE TSERS

Tourette Discussion for Kids
majordomo@chebucto.ns.ca
SUBSCRIBE TS-KIDS

Delirium, Dementia, and Amnestic and Other Cognitive Disorders

The disorders listed represent a clinically significant deficit in cognition or memory indicating a major change from a previous level of functioning. The disorders are:

A. Delirium, a disturbance of consciousness and a change in cognition developing over a short period of time.

B. Dementia, multiple cognitive deficits, including impairment in memory.

C. Amnestic Disorder, a memory impairment in the absence of other significant cognitive impairments.

A. *Delirium*

http://www.mentalhealth.com/dis1/p21-or01.html
Delirium: American Description
Diagnostic criteria, associated features, differential diagnosis.

http://www.mentalhealth.com/dis-rs3/p26-or01.html
Delirium: Research regarding Cause
Summary of research regarding causes of delirium.

http://www.mentalhealth.com/dis-rs1/p24-or01.html
Delirium: Research regarding Diagnosis
Summary of research studies regarding the diagnosis of delirium.

http://www.mentalhealth.com/dis-rs2/p25-or01.html
Delirium: Research regarding Treatment
Summary of research studies regarding treatment of delirium.

http://oncolink.upenn.edu/pdq/305472.html
Delirium
Interesting article from the National Cancer Institute. Discusses the relationship of organic mental disorders and cancer.

B. *Dementia*

i. ALZHEIMER'S TYPE

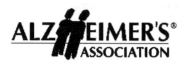

http://www.alz/org
Alzheimer's Association ★
Chicago, Illinois

Founded in 1980 the Association is the oldest and largest national voluntary health organization dedicated to research for the causes, cure, and prevention of Alzheimer's disease and to providing education and support services to Alzheimer's patients, their families and caregivers. Has more than 200 local chapters and several thousand support groups.

http://www.alzheimers.com/
Alzheimer's.com ★
NetHealth Inc.

Good all-purpose information site

http://www.cais.com/adear/adcdir.html
Alzheimer's Disease Center Directory ★

The National Institute on Aging funds 29 Alzheimer's Disease Centers. Research is underway to translate research advances into improved care and diagnosis of Alzheimer's patients while still focusing on the long-term goal of finding a method of prevention and cure for Alzheimer's. Hyperlinks to the 29 Alzheimer's Disease Centers.

http://www.alzheimers.org/adfact.html
Alzheimer's Disease: Fact Sheet ★

Discusses Alzheimer's symptoms, diagnosis, research, where to obtain more information.

http://weber.u.washington.edu/~adrcweb/
Alzheimer's Disease Research Center ★

Information on health care resources, educational resources and community support for patients and families. Major research areas: genetic analysis of AD subgroups; role of glucocorticoids in cognitive decline in aged monkeys; role of perlecan in pathogenesis of AD; development of transgenic mouse models based on overexpression of C-terminal domain of human APP; research on neurotropic effects of estrogens in aging brain. From the University of Washington.

Alzheimer's Disease REVIEW
ISSN 1093-5355   www.coa.uky.edu/ADReview
About ADR | Contents | Editorial Board | Register/Subscribe | Author
Info | Meetings | Jobs | Related Web Sites

http://www.coa.uky.edu/ADReview/
Alzheimer's Disease Review

Discusses latest advances in research on Alzheimer's and related disorders.

http://www.alzheimers.org/unravel.html
Alzheimer's Disease: Unraveling the Mystery ★

The National Institute on Aging and National Institutes of Health offer very comprehensive articles dealing with Alzheimer's disease; search for causes; research on diagnosis; investigating treatments; glossary. Contains many graphic representations of the brain.

http://www.biostat.wustl.edu/alzheimer/
Alzheimer's Page from Washington University ★
St. Louis, Missouri

Offers many references and hyperlinks to FAQ, current research, newest aging and dementia sites, a search of the Alzheimer's archives.

http://www.alzforum.org/
Alzheimer Research Forum

A non-profit organization established for the purpose of supporting the information needs of researchers and to promote openness and collaboration with colleagues worldwide to accelerate their common search for effective treatments for Alzheimer's disease.

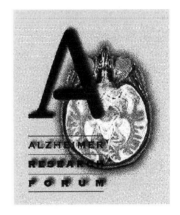

http://www.noah.cuny.edu/aging/aging.html
Ask NOAH About Aging and Alzheimer's Disease ★★

Primary source for information. Very comprehensive with many hyperlinks. Discusses aging; care and treatment of the elderly; aging information resources; Alzheimer's disease; Alzheimer's care and treatment; Alzheimer's research; other resources.

http://www.uokhsc.edu/sections/neuropath/cando.htm
Center for Alzheimer's and Neurodegenerative Disorders
Oklahoma City, Oklahoma

The Oklahoma City V.A. opened this center to serve as a regional and national model for treatment. A patient-focused and case management model of evaluation, treatment, and care is utilized in order to implement an innovative longitudinal model of care.

http://www.mentalhealth.com/mag1/p5m-alz3.html
Cognitive Tests 90% Accurate in Predicting Alzheimer's

Brief article from *Toronto Medical Post* indicating that cognitive tests are very accurate in predicting dementia of the Alzheimer type.

http://uhs.bsd.uchicago.edu/uhs/topics/delirium.dementia.html
Confusion in the Elderly

Discusses dementia, delirium and depression. Offers definition of syndromes; causes of delirium; how to conduct an examination; managing of a patient's delirium.

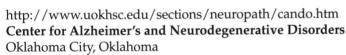

Confusion in the Elderly

http://www.cmhc.com/articles/adtest.htm
First Accurate Alzheimer's Test
> Discusses the accuracy of the AD7C(TM) test of Nymox. Helps doctors quickly rule out or diagnose Alzheimer's disease. More information may be found at <http://www.nymox .com>

http://www.alz.org/medical/ainar/1.html
Risk Factors for Alzheimer's Disease
> Discusses advances in Alzheimer's research, answering such questions are who is at risk, age at onset, family history, etc.

ii. VASCULAR DEMENTIA

http://www.med.harvard.edu/BWHRad/BrainSPECT/MID/MID.html
Multi-infarct (Vascular) Dementia ★
> By Holman, Chandak and Garada. Discusses history, images, findings, tutorial, a random case, slide-show, feedback and contents.

http://www.mentalhealth.com/dis1/p21-or02.html
Multi-infarct Dementia: American Description
> Diagnostic criteria, associated features, differential diagnosis.

http:///www.mentalhealth.com/dis-rs1/p24-or02.html
Multi-infarct Dementia: Research regarding Diagnosis
> Summary of research articles regarding diagnosis of multi-infarct dementia.

http://www.mentalhealth.com/dis-rs2/p25-or02.html
Multi-infarct Dementia: Research regarding Treatment
> Summary of research articles regarding treatment of multi-infarct dementia.

iii. HIV

http://www.yahoo.com/Health/Diseases_and_Conditions/AIDS_ HIV
AIDS/HIV ★
> Offers many links to AIDS/HIV, including organizations, programs, publications, research and treatment, support.

http://www.pslgroup.com/AIDS.HTM
AIDS/HIV: Doctor's Guide Information and Resources ★
> Links to current information regarding medical news and alerts.

- **Yahoo! Net Events: AIDS/HIV** - today's chats and programs.
- **Indices** (10)

- **Companies@**
- **Education** (74) NEW!
- **Events** (86) NEW!
- **General Information** (84)
- **HIV Antibody Testing** (7)
- **Hospice@**
- **Lesbian, Gay and Bisexual Resources** (32)
- **News** (16)

- **Organizations** (189) NEW!
- **Personal Experience** (42)
- **Prison Inmates** (11)
- **Programs** (13)
- **Publications** (14)
- **Research and Treatment** (84) NEW!
- **Support@**
- **Women** (2)
- **Usenet** (3)

Yahoo! Internet Life shows you the way to the best sites!
Click here to try it **Free**

http://www.teleport.com/~celinec/aids.shtml
AIDS Resource List ★
> Contains regional, national, and international sites.

http://www.cdcnac.org/
CDC National AIDS Clearinghouse ★
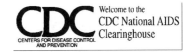
> Center for Disease Control's AIDS Clearinghouse's services are designed to facilitate the sharing of HIV/AIDS and STD resources and information about education and prevention, published materials, and research findings, as well as news about related trends.

iv. HEAD TRAUMA

No disorders solely related to this disorder appear on the Internet. This disorder may be included in articles dealing with disorders in general.

v. PARKINSON'S DISEASE

http://www.parkinsonsdisease.com/
Awakenings PD forum ★
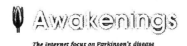
> An open forum for everyone involved with Parkinson's. Aims to increase dialogue among people with PD, carers, primary care physicians, and specialists in order to improve understanding and management of the condition.

http://www.cnsonline.org/www/archive/parkins/park-03.txt
Exercises for the Parkinson Patient
> Lists ten basic exercises for the Parkinson patient.

http://neurosurgery.mgh.harvard.edu/pd-suprt.htm
MGH/Harvard Guide to Organizations Providing Parkinson's Disease Support ★
> Comprehensive links to online information about Parkinson's disease. Lists the professional associations in various states and countries.

http://www.frostbyte.com/mulligan/parkinsons
Mulligan Foundation ★
Whitmore Lake, Michigan
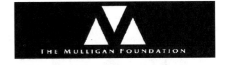
> Good resource. Foundation is dedicated to communicating technology, information and quality of life issues. Contains Parkinson's registry; Parkinson's profile; quality of life issues; research facilities; national organizations; support groups; and reciprocal links.

http://www.parkinson.org/
National Parkinson Foundation ★
Miami, Florida
> Foundation's mission is to find the cause and cure for Parkinson's and related neurodegenerative disorders through research; to educate medical practitioners to detect the early warning signs of Parkinson's; to educate patients, caregivers and the general public; to improve the quality of life for patients and caregivers.

http://demOnmac.mgh.harvard.edu/interactions$/forum/index
Neurology Webforums at MGH ★
> A continuing effort by Department of Neurology at MGH to foster interactive, online questions about various neurology-related topics.

http://neurosurgery.mgh.harvard.edu/pd-refs.htm
Pallidotomy Bibliography
> Reviews and summarizes articles dealing with pallidotomy and Parkinson's.

http://demOnmac.mgh.harvard.edu/newsletter/June1995/
pallidotomy.html
Pallidotomy for Parkinson's Disease
> Discusses symptoms and pallidotomy as a surgical treatment.

Parkinson's Digest
Parkinson's disease - Worldwide support group information exchange

http://www.harfordweb.com/pd/
Parkinson's Digest ★
> Not a source of medical information, but a reflection of how members of the Parkinson's community are coping with this condition. A worldwide support group information exchange.

http://www.cfn.cs.dal.ca/Health/NSPF/glossary.html
Parkinson Glossary of Terms
> Glossary of terms from A to Z.

http://neurosurgery.mgh.harvard.edu/pdstages.htm
Parkinson's Disease Staging ★
> Reference to Hoehn and Yahr's staging of Parkinson's disease. Goes through each stage in detailed fashion.

The Parkinson's Web http://pdweb.mgh.harvard.edu

http://pdweb.mgh.harvard.edu
Parkinson's Web ★
> Many hyperlinks to diagnosis and treatment of Parkinson's; recent research; surgical procedures; MGH Neurology Department; etc.

http://www.cnsonline.org/www/archive/parkins/park-01.txt
Special Report: Parkinson's Disease
> Excellent information on Parkinson's; treatment; blood-brain barrier; side effects of medications; research; dopamine agonist-blocking agents; research efforts; unsolved problems; problems with animal models.

vi. HUNTINGTON'S DISEASE

http://www.kumc.edu/hospital/huntingtons/
Caring for People With Huntington's Disease ★
> A site where patients, families, professionals can find help in caring for people with Huntington's disease. Contains articles on specific care issues as well as a listing of other sites related to Huntington's Disease.

http://neuro-chief-e.mgh.harvard.edu/mcmenemy/facinghd.html
Facing Huntington's Disease: Handbook ★
> Booklet copyrighted in Great Britain and published on the Massachusetts General Hospital site, contains chapters on medical facts; how HD is passed on; learning the diagnosis; young people at risk; course of illness; further sources of help.

http://neuro-www2.mgh.harvard.edu/hdsa/hdsamain.nclk
Huntington's Disease Society ★
New York, New York
> Information on Huntington's Disease Society of America (founded by Woody Guthrie's widow). Discusses Huntington's disease; issues of genetic testing; new research; research and fellowship grants; publications and videotapes.

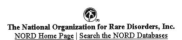

http://www.lib.uchicago.edu/~rd13/hd/outside.html
Internet Resources for Huntington's Disease ★
> Links to outside resources dealing with Huntington's disease.

vii. PICK'S DISEASE

http://www.ninds.nih.gov/healinfo/disorder/picks-picks.htm
Pick's Disease
National Institute of Health, Bethseda, Maryland
> Describes Pick's disease: treatment, prognosis, research, sources for more information.

http://www.stepstn.com/nord/rdb_sum/673.htm
Pick's Disease
> From the National Organization for Rare Disorders, describes all aspects of Pick's disease.

The National Organization for Rare Disorders, Inc.
NORD Home Page | Search the NORD Databases

◆ **Disease Information** ◆
Pick's Disease
ORDER FULL-TEXT VERSION | SUBSCRIBER SERVICE (password required)
Synonyms | Abstract (General Discussion) | Other Resources

http://count51.med.harvard.edu/BWHRad/BrainSPECT/Picks/Picks_Text.html
Pick's Disease (Lobar Atrophy)
> Describes the disease, pathological features, imaging, differential diagnosis and references.

viii. CREUTZFELDT-JAKOB DISEASE

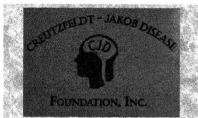

http://members.aol.com/crjakob/index.html
Creutzfeldt-Jakob Disease Foundation
North Miami, Florida
> The only American organization that focuses exclusively on Creutzfeldt-Jakob disease. Foundation seeks to promote the research, education, and awareness of CJD, as well as to reach out to people who have lost loved ones to this illness.

http://www.hrt.org/carecjd.html
Creutzfeldt-Jakob Mad Cow Disease Database ★
> Good source of articles and references.

3500+ articles on mad cow and Creutzfeldt-Jacob disease, prions, bovine spongiform encephalopathy, scrapie, BSE, CJD, CWD, TME, and TSE.
***Updated: 9 Dec 97* . . a project of the Sperling Biomedical Foundation**

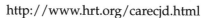

The Official Mad Cow Disease Home Page

http://www.mad-cow.org/
Official Mad Cow Disease Home Page ★
> A project of Sperling Biomedical Foundation, offers 3300+ articles on Mad Cow and Creutzfeldt-Jacob disease, prions, bovine spongiform encephalopathy, scrapie, BSE, CJD, CWD, TME, and TSE.

http://www.nmia.com/%7Emdibble/prion.html
Prion Diseases
> Comprehensive article by Stanley Prusiner, the first to identify the disease.

C. *Amnestic Disorders*

http://www.u.arizona.edu/~pdavidso/amcog.html
Amnesia and Cognition Unit, Department of Psychology
University of Arizona
> A neuropsychology research laboratory dedicated to studying memory and amnesia. Main focus is on explaining changes in memory due to aging and brain injury.

http://www.crc.nus.sg/CH/students/mce/psycho/amnesia.html
Amnestic Syndrome
> Discusses symptoms and signs; types; differential diagnosis; etiology and pathogenesis; treatment.

D. *Miscellaneous Dementia References*

http://www.mentalhealth.com/dis1/p21-or05.html
Dementia: American Description
> Presents diagnostic criteria, associated features, and differential diagnosis.

http://www.mentalhealth.com/dis1/p21-or03.html
Dementia Associated with Alcoholism
> Diagnostic criteria, associated features, differential diagnosis.

http://www.mentalhealth.com/dis-rs3/p26-or04.html
Dementia of the Alzheimer Type: Research regarding Cause
> Lengthy summary of research regarding the cause of dementia of the Alzheimer type.

http://www.mentalhealth.com/dis-rs1/p24-or04.html
Dementia of the Alzheimer Type: Research regarding Diagnosis
> Lengthy summary of research regarding the diagnosis of dementia of the Alzheimer type.

http://www.mentalhealth.com/dis-rs2/p25-or04.html
Dementia of the Alzheimer Type: Research regarding Treatment
> Lengthy summary of research regarding treatment for dementia of the Alzheimer type.

http://dementia.ion.ucl.ac.uk
Dementia Web ★
> Source of information, advice, education, research findings and support for patients, caregivers, doctors and other professionals.

Dementia Web

http://www.angelfire.com/tn/NursingHome/index.html
Nursing Home Information Site ★
> Excellent resource for long term care information. Half of all people in nursing homes suffer from some form of dementia.

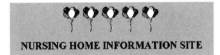

E. *Mailing Lists*

Alzheimer Discussion
majordomo@wubios.wustl.edu
SUBSCRIBE ALZHEIMER-DIGEST

Huntington's Disease
listserv@maelstrom.stjohns.edu
SUBSCRIBE HUNT-DIS

SECTION III.
Mental Disorders due to a General Medical Condition Not Elsewhere Classified

No articles solely related to these disorders are found on the Internet. These disorders may be included in articles dealing with disorders in general.

Substance~Related Disorders

Substance-Related Disorders refer to abuse of a drug, a medication, or a toxin. The substances are grouped into eleven classes:

A. Alcohol-Related Disorders
B. Amphetamine-Related Disorders
C. Caffeine-Related Disorders
D. Cannabis-Related Disorders
E. Cocaine-Related Disorders
F. Hallucinogen-Related Disorders
G. Inhalant-Related Disorders
H. Nicotine-Related Disorders
I. Opioid-Related Disorders
J. Phencyclidine-Related Disorders
K. Sedative-Related Disorders

A. Alcohol~Related Disorders

DIAGNOSIS, TREATMENT, AND RESEARCH

http://www.mentalhealth.com/dis1/p21-sb01.html
Alcohol Dependence: American Description
Diagnostic criteria, associated features, differential diagnosis.

http://www.mentalhealth.com/dis-rs3/p26-sb01.html
Alcohol Dependence: Research regarding Cause
Over one hundred pages of summaries of research regarding the cause of alcohol dependency.

http://www.mentalhealth.com/dis-rs1/p24-sb01.html
Alcohol Dependence: Research regarding Diagnosis
Almost 60 pages of summaries of research regarding the diagnosis of alcohol dependency.

http://www.mentalhealth.com/dis-rs2/p25-sb01.html
Alcohol Dependency: Research regarding Treatment
Over 50 pages of summaries of research regarding the treatment of alcohol dependency.

http://www.mentalhealth.com/rx/p23-sb01.html
Alcohol Dependence: Treatment
Medical treatments and psychosocial treatments.

Alcohol Dependence

Treatment

INTERNET
Mental Health

http://www.mentalhealth.com/mag1/p5h-al10.html
Alcohol Dependence: Treatment of Alcoholism
> From the *Harvard Mental Health Letter.* Provides a good overview of treatment issues.

http://www.cmhc.com/disorders/sx16.htm
Alcohol/Substance Dependence: Symptoms
> Lists *DSM-IV* criteria.

http://www.mentalhealth.com/mag1/p5m-alc1.html
Asking about Injuries May Help Reveal Drinking Problems
> Interesting article encouraging physicians to ask how frequently patients injure themselves rather than how much they drink.

http://www.drugs.indiana.edu/publications/ncadi/primer/binge.htm
Binge Drinking
> From Indiana Prevention Resource Center at Indiana University. Discusses binge drinking, factors involved, and prevention strategies.

http://kpix.com/xtra/keane/QA-19Dec-101450-L.html
Drunk Driving: 10 Questions and Answers regarding Law
> From KPIX legal analyst Peter Keane. Discusses California laws for drunk driving as well as some of the differences in other states.

Indiana Prevention Resource Center

FactLine

on Alcohol Doses, Measurements, and Blood Alcohol Levels

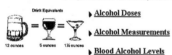

▸ Alcohol Doses
▸ Alcohol Measurements
▸ Blood Alcohol Levels

http://www.drugs.indiana.edu/publications/iprc/factline/alcdoses.html
Factline on Alcohol Doses, Measurements, and Blood Alcohol Levels
> From the Indiana Prevention Resource Center. Discusses alcohol doses, alcohol measurements, blood alcohol levels.

http://www.drugs.indiana.edu/publications/iprc/factline/lowalc.html
Factline on Very-Low Alcohol Beverages
> From the Indiana Prevention Resource Center. Offers good information on non-alcoholic brews.

http://www.mentalhealth.com/mag1/p5h-fas1.html
Fetal Alcohol Syndrome
> From the *Harvard Mental Health Letter.* Discusses the devastating effects of FAS.

http://www.mentalhealth.com/dx/dx-sb01.html
Online Diagnosis
> Reviews criteria for psychiatric diagnosis. Also contains a questionnaire to aid with diagnosis.

http://www.mentalhealth.com/mag1/p5m-dr01.html
Prescription Drugs and Alcohol Too Often Lethal Mix
> Comments on research study from Toronto indicating that pre-scription drugs and over-the-counter medications play a leading role in road accidents.

http://www.recovery.org/acoa/acoa.1.html
Research on Children of Alcoholics
> This Alcohol Alert focuses on three major research questions concerning COAs: (1) What contributes to resilience in some COAs? (2) Do COAs differ from children of nonalcoholics? (3) Are the differences related to parental alcoholism?

http://www.ovchin.uc.edu/htdocs/alcoholtest.html
What Are the Signs of Alcoholism?
> The NCADD self-test intended to help determine if you or someone you know needs to find out more about alcoholism.

What are the Signs of Alcoholism?

THe NCADD self-test

Here is a self-test to help you review the role alcohol plays in your life. These questions incorporate many of the common symptoms of alcoholism. This test is intended to help you determine if you or someone you know needs to find out more about alcoholism; it is not intended to be used to establish the diagnosis of alcoholism.

RESOURCES WITH SPECIAL RELEVANCE TO ALCOHOLISM

http://www.alcoholics-anonymous.org/factfile/aafactfi.html
A.A. Fact File ★
> Provides basic information about AA. Contains sections and links on such topics as: how to contact A.A.; membership; structure; 12 Steps; AA traditions; AA and alcoholism; anonymity; public relationships; AA meetings; literature and audiovisual materials; historical data; locations outside the US and Canada.

http://www.gate.net/%7Esmulder/rec/pages/toc.html
ACA Online Meeting Manual
> Contains many links to finding meetings; letter to a newcomer; the solution; serenity prayer; FAQ; and many more.

http://www.al-anon.org/
Al-Anon and Alateen Homepage
> Al-Anon is a program of recovery based on 12 Steps, 12 Traditions, and 12 Concepts of Service adopted from AA. Contains sections and links on: how to find help anywhere in the world; questions to help determine whether you are affected by someone else's drinking; information on the 12- Step traditions and concepts; books and pamphlets. Also available in Spanish.

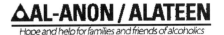

http://www.iugm.org/av/
Alcoholics Victorious
Kansas City. Missouri

> Founded in 1948, AV support groups offer a safe environment where recovering people who recognize Jesus Christ as their "Higher Power"can gather together and share their experience, strength, and hope. The 12-Steps and Alcoholics Victorious Creed are used at most meetings.

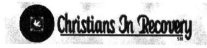

http://www.christians-in-recovery.com/
Christians in Recovery

> CIR helps people regain and maintain balance and order in their lives through active discussion of the 12-Steps, the Bible, and experiences in their own recovery.

http://www.geocities.com/Paris/3733/links.html
Co-dependency Links ★

> Contains links to recovery pages with information about co-dependency; news groups about co-dependency and related issues; Internet relay chat information; organizations with information about co-dependency.

http://www.jacsweb.org/
Jewish Alcoholics Chemically Dependent and Significant Others

> Online recovery magazine for Jews and their families whose lives have been affected by alcohol and drug abuse, and for rabbis and treatment professionals concerned with chemical dependency in the Jewish community.

http://comnet.org/mm/
Moderation Management

> MM is a recovery program for people who have made the decision to reduce their drinking and make other positive lifestyle changes. Discusses balance, moderation, self-management, personal responsibility.

http://www.madd.org/
Mothers Against Drunk Driving ★
Dallas, Texas

> Moms, dads, and others determined to stop drunk driving and to support victims of this violent crime. Contains information on how to become a member, how to find a local chapter, statistics, supporting MADD, other links.

http://www.naadac.org/
National Association on Alcoholism and Drug Abuse Counselors ★
Arlington, Virginia

> Founded in 1972, NAADAC's mission is to provide leadership in the alcoholism and drug abuse counseling profession by building new visions, effecting change in public policy, promoting criteria for effective treatment, encouraging adherence to ethical standards, and ensuring professional growth for alcoholism and drug abuse counselors.

http://www.ncadd.org/
National Council on Alcoholism and Drug Dependence ★
New York, New York

> Founded in 1944, NCADD is a voluntary health organization with a nationwide network of affiliates. Advocates prevention, intervention, research, and treatment and is dedicated to ridding the disease of its stigma and its sufferers from denial and shame.

http://www.recovery.org/aa/
Online AA Resources ★

> Contains hyperlinks to everything you need to know about AA. Also includes non-English AA resources and AA literature.

http://www.health.org/
Prevention Online ★

> From U.S. National Clearinghouse for Alcohol and Drug Information, offers electronic access to searchable databases and substance abuse prevention materials that pertain to alcohol, tobacco, and other drugs.

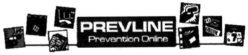

A service of SAMHSA

	Alcohol & Drug Facts	
What's New	Search PREVLINE & Other Sites	Publications/Catalog
Resources & Referrals		Online Forums
Research & Statistics		Conference Calendar
Searchable Databases	NEWSROOM	Related Internet Links
Campaigns	UPDATED DAILY	Dynatable

http://www.rational.org/recovery/Q%26A.html
Rational Recovery

> Discusses Rational Recovery as an alternative to traditional 12-Step programs and group meetings.

http://www.recovering-couples.org/
Recovering Couples Anonymous ★

> Offers a 12-Step program that includes tools for developing mature, healthy relationships.

http://www.sobervacations.com/
Sober Vacations International

> Specializing in vacations for recovering alcoholics and others in recovery.

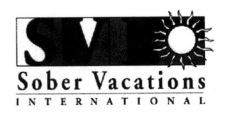

http://www.winternet.com/~terrym/sobriety.html

Sobriety and Recovery Resources ★★

> Very large resource that offers many hyperlinks to every facet of sobriety and recovery. A must for people working in the field.

http://www.pilot.infi.net/~susanf/acapoint.htm

Un-official ACOA Page

> Explains typical characteristics and problems many adults find in later life after having grown up in an alcoholic or otherwise dysfunctional home. Many links.

http://www.mediapulse.com/wfs/

Women for Sobriety ★

Quakertown, Pennsylvania

> Providing services to women alcoholics since 1976, WOS is both an organization and a self-help program for women alcoholics. It offers a "New Life" Program based on a 13- statement program of positivity that encourages emotional and spiritual growth.

B. *Amphetamine-Related Disorders*

http://www.mentalhealth.com/dis1/p21-sb02.html

Amphetamine Dependence: American Description

> Diagnostic criteria, associated features, and differential diagnosis.

http://www.mentalhealth.com/dx/dx-sb02.html

Amphetamine Dependence: Online Diagnosis

> Gives criteria needed for accurate psychiatric diagnosis. Also offers an online screening to aid in diagnosis.

http://www.mentalhealth.com/rx/p23-sb02.html

Amphetamine Dependence: Treatment

> Medical and psychosocial treatments.

http://www.mentalhealth.com/dis-rs3/p26-sb02.html

Amphetamine Dependence: Research regarding Cause

> Summary of research dealing with the cause of amphetamine dependence.

http://www.mentalhealth.com/dis-rs1/p24-sb02.html

Amphetamine Dependence: Research regarding Diagnosis

> Summary of research dealing with diagnosis of amphetamine dependence.

Amphetamine Dependence

Research Re: Treatment

http://www.mentalhealth.com/dis-rs2/p25-sb02.html

Amphetamine Dependence: Research regarding Treatment

> Summary of several articles dealing with research in the treatment of amphetamine dependence.

http://www.lec.org/DrugSearch/Documents/Amphetamines
.html
Amphetamines Fact Sheet
> Quick overview including slang terms, immediate effects and behaviors.

http://www.hyperreal.com/drugs/e4x/
E For Ecstasy
> Discusses history of ecstasy; what it does and how it works; who takes the drug; dangers; the law; other uses of ecstasy.

http://www.drugs.indiana.edu/pubs/factline/ampet.html
Factline on Amphetamines
> From Indiana Prevention Resource Center at Indiana University. Discusses "look-alike" drugs, methamphetamines, "Crystal," "Ice," "Glass," legal issues.

C. *Caffeine~Related Disorders*

http://www.uiuc.edu/departments/mckinley/health-info/
drug-alc/caffeine.html
Caffeine
> Discusses the general effects of caffeine, effects on performance, problems with energizing, health risks, quitting the habit, resources.

D. *Cannabis~Related Disorders*

http://marijuana-as-medicine.org/
Alliance for Cannabis Therapeutics
Washington, D.C.
> Founded in 1981, ACT concentrates solely on the question of marijuana's medical utility and has no policy regarding the nonmedical use of cannabis. ACT's goal is to end the federal prohibition of cannabis in medicine.

information about
medical uses of marijuana
clinical studies
reform efforts

This site has been accessed
020837
times since 01/01/97.
Thank you! Come again!

What do you think about voter initiatives?

http://www.mentalhealth.com/dis1/p21-sb03.html
Cannabis Dependence: American Description
> Diagnostic criteria, associated features, differential diagnosis.

http://www.mentalhealth.com/dx/dx-sb03.html
Cannabis Dependence: Online Diagnosis
> Gives criteria needed for accurate psychiatric diagnosis. Also offers an online screening as an aid to diagnosis.

http://www.mentalhealth.com/dis-rs3/p26-sb03.html
Cannabis Dependence: Research regarding Cause
> Summaries of research articles regarding cause of cannabis dependence.

http://www.mentalhealth.com/dis-rs1/p24-sb03.html
Cannabis Dependence: Research regarding Diagnosis
Summaries of research articles regarding diagnosis of cannabis dependence.

http://www.mentalhealth.com/dis-rs2/p25-sb03.html
Cannabis Dependence: Research regarding Treatment
Summaries of research articles regarding the treament of cannabis dependence.

http://www.mentalheatlh.com/rx/p23-sb03.html
Cannabis Dependence: Treatment
Medical and psychosocial treatments.

http://www.mentalhealth.com/mag1/p5m-sb01.html
For Potheads, Brain Remains Impaired Long After the Buzz is Gone
Describes research at Harvard concluding that heavy use is associated with residual neuropsychological effects even after one day of supervised abstinence from the drug.

http://raru.adelaide.edu.au/T95/paper/s1p2.html
Marijuana's Effects on Actual Driving Performance
From the Netherlands, this article describes the results of a research program that was set up to determine the dose reponse relationship between marijuana and objectively and subjectively measured aspects of real world driving.

 Welcome To The Marijuana Anonymous Home Page!

What Is Marijuana Anonymous?

Marijuana Anonymous is a fellowship of men and women who share our experience, strength, and hope with each other that we may solve our common problem and help others to recover from marijuana addiction.

http://www.marijuana-anonymous.org/
Marijuana Anonymous Home Page
A fellowship of men and women who share experiences, strength, and hope with each other in order to solve common problems and help others recover from marijuana addiction. Uses the basic 12-Steps of Recovery founded by AA.

http://www.calyx.net/~olsen/MEDICAL/
Marijuana as a Medicine ★
Hyperlinks to state and national legislation; court rulings and filings; medical journals and other publications; state and national media; etc.

http://www.mentalhealth.com/book/p45-mari.html
Marijuana: Facts for Teens
Answers to questions teens might have regarding usage; why young people begin to smoke; how marijuana affects school, sports, driving, and other activities; etc.

http://www.mentalhealth.com/book/p45-mar2.html
Marijuana: Facts Parents Need to Know
>Many hyperlinks to questions parents have about marijuana and their children. Wonderful for parents and professionals working in the field.

E. *Cocaine-Related Disorders*

http://www.ca.org/whatisca.html
Cocaine Anonymous
>A fellowship of men and women who share their experience, strength, and hope with each other so that they can solve their common problem and help others to recover from their addiction.

Cocaine Anonymous
World Services
"We're Here and We're Free"

http://www.ca.org/test.html
Cocaine Anonymous: Self-Test for Cocaine Addiction
>A 23-item test. A "yes" answer to any one of these may indicate that a person has a cocaine problem.

http://www.mentalhealth.com/dx/dx-sb04.html
Cocaine Dependence: Online Diagnosis
>Gives criteria needed for accurate psychiatric diagnosis. Also offers an online screening to aid in diagnosis.

http://www.mentalhealth.com/dis1/p21-sb04.html
Cocaine Dependence: American Description
>Diagnostic criteria, associated features, differential diagnosis

http://www.mentalhealth.com/dis-rs3/p26-sb04.html
Cocaine Dependence: Research regarding Cause
>Summary of dozens of research articles dealing with the cause of cocaine dependence.

http://www.mentalhealth.com/dis-rs1/p24-sb04.html
Cocaine Dependence: Research regarding Diagnosis
>Summary of many research articles dealing with the diagnosis of cocaine dependence.

http://www.mentalhealth.com/dis-rs2/p25-sb04.html
Cocaine Dependence: Research regarding Treatment
>Summary of many research articles with the treatment of cocaine dependence.

http://www.mentalhealth.com/rx/p23-sb04.html
Cocaine Dependence: Treatment
>Reviews medical and psychosocial treatments

http://www.noah.cuny.edu/pregnancy/march_of_dimes/
substance/cocaine.html
Cocaine Use during Pregnancy
Good article reviewing effects of cocaine use on unborn babies. Describes problems faced by babies whose mothers used cocaine during pregnancy.

Public information materials are available in print form from the ARF Marketing Services (Telephone 1-800-661-1111, 416-595-6059; fax 416-593-4694). Reduced prices will be offered to Ontario government-funded agencies and on large volume orders.

www.arf.org/isd/pim/cocaine.html ❶ Copyright ARF 1995

FACTS ABOUT...COCAINE

http://www.arf.org/isd/pim/cocaine.html
Facts about Cocaine
From Addiction Research Foundation. Reviews information on cocaine as a central nervous system stimulant.

F. *Hallucinogen-Related Disorders*

http://www.mentalhealth.com/dis1/p21-sb05.html
Hallucinogen Dependence: American Description
Diagnostic criteria, associated features and differential diagnosis.

http://www.mentalhealth.com/dx/dx-sb05.html
Hallucinogen Dependence: Online Diagnosis
Gives criteria needed for accurate psychiatric diagnosis. Also offers an online screening as an aid to diagnosis.

http://www.mentalhealth.com/dis-rs1/p24-sb05.html
Hallucinogen Dependence: Research
Summary of research articles dealing with hallucinogen dependence.

http://www.mentalhealth.com/rx/p23-sb05.html
Hallucinogen Dependence: Treatment
Medical and psychosocial treatments.

http://www.fda.gov/fdac/features/795_psyche.html
Medical Possibilities for Psychedelic Drugs
The FDA has sought ways to allow human studies to test for psychedelic drugs to determine usefulness. This concept and conclusions are discussed.

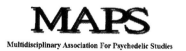

Multidisciplinary Association For Psychedelic Studies

http://www.maps.org/
Multidisciplinary Association for Psychedelic Studies ★
Charlotte, North Carolina
MAPS focuses on the development of beneficial, socially-sanctioned use of psychedelic drugs and marijuana. MAPS helps scientific researchers design, obtain government approval for, fund, and conduct and report on psychedelic research in human volunteers.

http://www.calyx.com/~schaffer/lsd/lsdmenu.html
Psychedelic Library ★
    Research papers and monographs concerning the several uses of psychedelic drugs in the treatment of addictions, personality disorders and other conditions. Hyperlinks to many other topics dealing with psychedelics.

http://www.drugtext.nl/library/psychedelics/thermenu.html
Psychotherapy and Psychedelic Drugs ★
    Hyperlinks to various papers dealing with psychotherapy and psychedelic drugs. Most are old but can be useful.

G. *Inhalant~Related Disorders*

http://www.drugs.indiana.edu/pubs/factline/inhal.html
Factline on Inhalants
    Discusses inhalants, warning signs of inhalant use, common inhalants, effects of inhalant use, effects of inhalant intoxication, parent/teacher alert, legal issues, pattern of use.

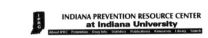

Indiana Prevention Resource Center

FactLine

on Inhalants

http://www.jointogether.org/jto/issues/inhalants/inhalant_index.stm
Inhalant Abuse
    An overview of inhalant abuse, list of warning signs, fact sheet summarizing dangers and national trends, action steps.

http://www.mentalhealth.com/rx/p23-sb06.html
Inhalant Dependence: Treatment
    Medical and psychosocial treatments.

http://www.drugs.indiana.edu/pubs/radar/rguides/inhalan.html
Resource Guide: Inhalants
    Comprehensive resource guide regarding inhalants.

H. *Nicotine~Related Disorders*

http://www.ash.org/
Action on Smoking and Health Web Page ★
Washington, D.C.
    A national legal-action antismoking organization in existence for 30 years. Supported solely by contributions. Web pages contains dozens of current articles dealing with all aspects of nicotine.

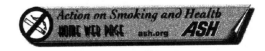

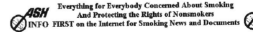

http://www.clever.net/chrisco/nosmoke/lastcig.html
After the Last Cigarette
    Gives physiological and psychological changes after minutes, days, weeks, and months of not smoking.

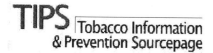

TIPS Tobacco Information & Prevention Sourcepage

http://www.cdc.gov/tobacco/
Center for Disease Control's Tobacco Information and Prevention Page ★

Everything you want to know about nicotine. Presents Surgeon General's report, research, tips on quitting, educational materials, FAQ, resources.

http://www.kickbutt.org/
Kickbutt.Org
Seattle, Washington

A non-profit health promotion organization founded in 1982, inspired by DOC (Doctors Ought to Care), Kickbutt attempts to link different tobacco control groups, improve access to vital information, and provide communities with the necessary tools to work for change.

The Master Anti-Smoking Page

    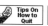 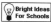

http://www.autonomy.com/smoke.htm
Master Anti-Smoking Page ★

Designed to help people quit smoking. Contains links to every anti-smoking page on the web. Special section for people doing research as well as tips for quitting smoking.

http://rampages.onramp.net/~nica/
Nicotine Anonymous ★

Fellowship of people helping each other quit smoking and lead lives free from nicotine. Opportunity to share experience, strength, and offer hope. Only membership requirement is the desire to stop using nicotine.

http://tobacco.arizona.edu
Nicotine and Tobacco Network ★

Contains links to a tobacco library, nicotine and tobacco news, kids and tobacco, research updates, pro-tobacco point of view, tobacco and disease, Arizona activities.

http://www.mentalhealth.com/dis1/p21-sb07.html
Nicotine Dependence: American Description

Diagnostic criteria, associated features, differential diagnosis.

http://www.mentalhealth.com/dx/dx-sb07.html
Nicotine Dependence: Online Diagnosis

Gives criteria needed for accurate psychiatric diagnosis. Also offers an online screening as an aid to diagnosis.

http://www.mentalhealth.com/rx/p23-sb07.html
Nicotine Dependence Treatment

Medical and psychosocial treatments.

http://www.mentalhealth.com/dis-rs3/p26-sb07.html
Nicotine Dependence: Research regarding Cause
> Summary of research articles dealing with cause of nicotine dependence.

http://www.mentalhealth.com/dis-rs1/p24-sb07.html
Nicotine Dependence: Research regarding Diagnosis
> Summary of research articles dealing with diagnosis of nicotine dependence.

http://www.mentalhealth.com/dis-rs2/p25-sb07.html
Nicotine Dependence: Research regarding Treatment
> Summary of research articles dealing with treatment of nicotine dependence.

http://home1.gte.net/kclement/qstoday/index.htm
> **Quit Smoking Today!** ★
> Dedicated to helping quit smoking, site contains three sections: (1) list of important facts and statistics related to smoking; (2) list of organizations providing current information, advice and suggestions; (3) list of links to pages dedicated to people who want to stop smoking.

http://www.tobacco.org/Documents/9406EPA.html
Secondhand Smoke Is a Preventable Health Risk
> From the U. S. Environmental Protection Agency. This article comments on a report that concluded that secondhand smoke causes lung cancer in adult nonsmokers and impairs the respiratory health of children.

http://www.mentalhealth.com/mag1/p5h-smk1.html
Smoking and Depression: New Data
> From the *Harvard Mental Health Letter*. Explores the issue of why people addicted to alcohol, cocaine, heroin, and other drugs are known to have a high rate of depression.

http://www.clc.upmc.edu:80/CLC_HTML/smoking.html
Smoking Cessation
> From the Comprehensive Lung Center at the University of Pittsburgh Medical Center. Presents the stages of the behavioral process of smoking as well as many good reasons to stop smoking.

http://www.tobacco.org/
Tobacco BBS Resource Center ★★
> A resource center focusing on tobacco and smoking issues. Features tobacco news, information assistance for smokers trying to quit, alerts for tobacco control advocates, open debate on issues of tobacco, nicotine, cigarettes and cigars.

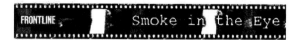

Tobacco on the WWW

http://www.pbs.org/wgbh/pages/frontline/smoke/links/
Tobacco on the Web ★
> From WGBH, Boston, Educational Foundation, site links are broken into three sections: (1) general information tobacco sites; (2) specific focus sites; (3) how to quit sites.

http://www.ahsc.arizona.edu/nicnet/sympcope.htm
Withdrawal Symptoms: What to Expect
> Lengthy article listing symptoms, their causes, and ways to obtain relief.

I. *Opioid-Related Disorders*

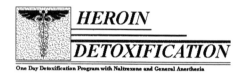

One Day Detoxification Program with Naltrexone and General Anesthesia

http://www.heroin-detox.com/
Heroin Detoxification: One Day
> Serves as a base for education, promotion, and discussion related to naltrexone-induced heroin detoxification under general anesthesia.

http://www.mentalhealth.com/mag1/p5h-sb03.html
Lessons from the Vietnam Heroin Experience
> From the *Harvard Mental Health Letter*. Describes research data from Vietnam veterans. Results indicated that more men had been using opiates in Vietnam than the Department of Defense had thought.

Welcome to the **National Alliance of Methadone Advocates** WWW Site

http://www.methadone.org/
National Alliance of Methadone Advocates ★
New York, New York
> An organization of methadone maintenance patients and supporters of quality methadone maintenance treatments. Promotes methadone maintenance treatment as the most effective modality for the treatment of heroin addiction.

http://www.mentalhealth.com/dis1/p21-sb08.html
Opioid Dependence: American Description
> Diagnostic criteria necessary to diagnose opioid dependency.

http://www.mentalhealth.com/dx/fdx-sb08.html
Opioid Dependence Diagnosis
> Criteria necessary for accurate psychiatric diagnosis.

http://www.mentalhealth.com/dis-rs3/p26-sb08.html
Opioid Dependence: Research regarding Cause
> Summary of research articles dealing with the cause of opioid dependence.

http://www.mentalhealth.com/dis-rs1/p24-sb08.html
Opioid Dependence: Research regarding Diagnosis
> Summary of research articles dealing with diagnosis of opioid dependence.

http://www.mentalhealth.com/dis-rs2/p25-sb08.html
Opioid Dependence: Research regarding Treatment
> Summary of research articles dealing with treatment of opioid dependence.

http://www.mentalhealth.com/rx/p23-sb08.html
Opioid Dependence: Treatment
> Medical and psychosocial treatments.

J. *Phencyclidine-Related Disorders*

http://www.nida.nih.gov/NIDACapsules/NCPCP.html
Phencyclidine
> From the National Institute on Drug Abuse. Discusses PCP usage and health hazards.

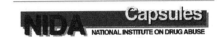

PCP (Phencyclidine)

http://www.mentalhealth.com/dis1/p21-sb09.html
Phencyclidine Dependence: American Description
> Diagnostic criteria, associated features, and differential diagnosis.

http://www.mentalhealth.com/dx/fdx-sb09.html
Phencyclidine Dependence Diagnosis
> Criteria necessary for accurate psychiatric diagnosis.

http://www.mentalhealth.com/dis-rs1/p24-sb09.html
Phencyclidine Dependence: Research
> Several research articles dealing with phencyclidine dependence.

http://www.mentalhealth.com/rx/p23-sb09.html
Phencyclidine Dependence: Treatment
> Medical and psychosocial treatments.

http://mentalhealth.com/mag1/p5h-sb06.html
Psychedelic Drugs
> Article from *Harvard Mental Health Letter*. Describes all aspects of psychedelic drugs.

K. *Sedative-Related Disorders*

http://www.erowid.com/entheogens/ghb/ghb.shtml
GHB ★
> Information on uses and abuses of GHB.

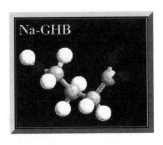

http://web.bu.edu/COHIS/subsabse/subsabse.htm (use menu)
Hypnotics and Sedative Abuse
> Discusses what hypnotic/sedative abuse is, where it comes from, how many people use hypnotics and sedatives, problem of abuse, morbidity and mortality statistics.

http://web.bu.edu/COHIS/subsabse/subsabse.htm (use menu)
Methaqualone and Other Hypnotic/Sedative Look-Alikes.
> Discusses methaqualone; hypnotic/sedative look-alikes; hypnotic/sedative abuse; signs and symptoms; treatments; prevention. Also contains a substance abuse menu.

http://www.usdoj.gov/dea/pubs/rohypnol/rohypnol.htm
Rohypnol
> Information from Drug Enforcement Administration. Sometimes called "date-rape" drug.

http://www.mentalhealth.com/dx/dx-sb10.html
Sedative Dependence: Online Diagnosis
> Gives criteria needed for accurate psychiatric diagnosis. Also offers an online screening as an aid to diagnosis.

http://www.mentalhealth.com/rx/p23-sb10.html
Sedative Dependence: Treatment
> Reviews medical treatment of barbiturate dependence, medical treatment of benzodiazepine dependence, psychosocial treatments.

L. *Miscellaneous Substance-Related Disorders*

http://www.teleport.com/~acudetox/GP/acuindex.html
Acupuncture in Recovery ★
> Many links to various sites explaining acupuncture for addiction.

http://www.wemac.com/hpaddict.html
Addiction in Health Professionals
> Lists characteristics and behaviors for alcohol as the drug of choice as well as when other drugs are used.

http://www.arf/org/
Addiction Research Foundation ★
Ontario, Canada
> Foundation's mission is to work with partners to create and apply knowledge to prevent and reduce harm associated with alcohol, tobacco and other drugs in Ontario communities.

http://www.atforum.com/index.html
Addiction Treatment Forum ★

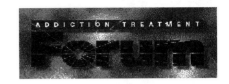

Designed to serve the addiction treatment community, the forum reports what has happened, what is happening today, and what might happen to further the successful treatment of drug addictions. Primary focus is opiate addiction and the benefits of methadone treatment.

http://www.winternet.com/~webpage/adolrecovery.html
Adolescence Substance Abuse and Recovery Resources ★

Teen-oriented links to useful resources. Good for parents, adolescents and mental health workers.

http://www.alcoholconcern.org.uk/
Alcohol Concern ★

London

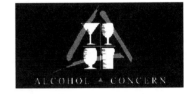

A national agency on alcohol misuse in England and Wales that wants to reduce the costs of alcohol misuse and develop the range and quality of helping services available to problem drinkers and their families.

http://www.aamro.com/
American Association of Medical Review Officers

Research Triangle Park, North Carolina

A non-profit medical board which has established national standards and certification for medical practitioners in the field of drug and alcohol testing.

http://www.holistic.com/ayurveda/addict01.htm
Ayurveda and Recovery From Addictions

A holistic approach, Ayurveda is used with persons who sincerely want to recover yet have problems with withdrawal. The article claims that Ayurveda not only helps remove the cause of addictions, but helps evaporate toxins so as to minimize withdrawal symptoms.

http://www.alcoholfreekids.com/
The Campaign for Alcohol Free Kids

Clearwater Beach, Florida

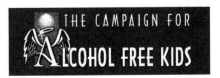

A national U.S. organization. CAFK offers email updates on alcohol-related topics.

http://www.ccsa.ca/
Canadian Centre on Substance Abuse ★

Ottawa

This non-profit organization works to minimize the harm associated with the use of alcohol, tobacco, and other drugs. Valuable hyperlinks.

http://www.caron.org/
The Caron Foundation
Wernersville, Pennsylvania
  Non-profit treatment for adolescents and adults

http://www.wemac.com/cdconcpt.html
Chemical Dependence: Current Concepts
  By West Michigan Addiction Consultants in Grand Rapids, Michigan. Offers links explaining what chemical dependency is, how it is recognized, what should be done once addiction is recognized, how family is affected, what is recovery, role of the physician.

http://printing.presstar.com/cda/
Chemically Dependent Anonymous Homepage
  Like AA, based on 12-Step program.

http://www.dare-america.com/
DARE
  DARE (Drug Abuse Resistance Education) is a site designed especially for kids. Contains links for kids, educators, parents, other news, officers, etc.

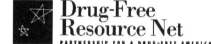

http://www.drugfreeamerica.org/
Drug-Free Resource Net ★
  From Partnership for a Drug-Free America. This site offers a comprehensive database regarding drugs, FAQ, help for parents, etc.

http://www.erols.com/ksciacca/
Dual Diagnosis Website ★
  Dual diagnosis is defined as co-occuring mental illness, drug addiction, and/or alcoholism. This site is designed to provide information and resources for service providers, consumers, and family members who are seeking assistance and/or education in this field.

http://www.arf.org/isd/bib/elderly.html
Elderly and Substance Abuse
  A bibliography containing references to articles dealing with substance abuse and the elderly.

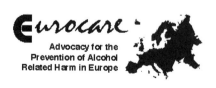
Advocacy for the Prevention of Alcohol Related Harm in Europe

http://www.eurocare.org/
Eurocare ★
London
  Advocacy for the prevention of alcohol-related harm in Europe. Offers information regarding alcohol in over twenty European countries.

http://www.bettyfordcenter.org/
The Betty Ford Center
Rancho Mirage, California
> A not-for-profit 12-Step treatment program.

http://www.cts.com/crash/habtsmrt/
Habit Smart
> Constructed to provide an abundance of information about addictive behavior: theories of habit endurance and habit change as well as tips for effectively managing problematic habitual behavior.

http://www.hazelden.org/
The Hazelden Foundation ★
Center City, Minnesota
> An online bookstore with many recovery resources.

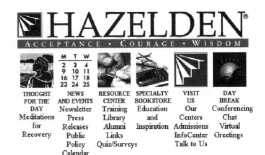

http://www.ibogaine.org/
Ibogaine Dossier ★
> Ibogaine is a substance discovered in plants from the West African rain forests reported to reduce both narcotic and cocaine withdrawal symptoms. Contains information for clinicians, patients, and those interested in NDA's ibogaine training symposia.

http://www.drugs.indiana.edu
Indiana Prevention Resource Center ★★
Indiana University
> Clearinghouse for prevention, technical assistance and information about alcohol, tobacco, and other drugs. Links to articles of national interest, legislative updates, job listings, etc.

http://www.drugfreeworkplace.org/
Institute for a Drug-Free Workplace
Washington, D.C.
> An independent, self-sustaining coalition of businesses, organizations, and individuals dedicated to preserving the rights of employers and employees in drug-abuse prevention programs and to positively influence the national debate on these issues.

http://www.jointogether.org/
Join Together Online ★
> A national resource center and meeting place for communities working to reduce substance abuse and gun violence.

http://www.lindesmith.org/
Lindesmith Center ★★
New York, New York
> A policy research institute featuring full-text articles from the academic and popular press focusing on drug policy from economic, criminal justice, and public health perspectives.

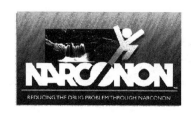

http://www.narconon.org/
Narconon Home Page
> A treatment program dealing with detoxification.

http://www.netwizards.net/recovery/na/
Narcotics Anonymous Home Page ★
> Started in 1947, NA is a society of recovering drug addicts. Contains invaluable hyperlinks to all aspects of NA.

http://www.iop.bpmf.ac.uk/home/depts/psychiat/nac/nac.html
National Addiction Center
London
> Established in 1991, NAC is a network of clinicians, researchers and clinical teachers sharing a commitment to excellence in work directed at the prevention and treatment of substance misuse, and to the support and strengthening of national and international endeavors in this field.

http://www.collection_sites.org
National Association of Collection Sites
Alexandria, Virginia
> Founded in September, 1995, as the industry trade association for sites performing drug and alcohol specimen collections.

http://www.casacolumbia.org/
The National Center on Addiction and Substance Abuse at Columbia University ★★
> CASA describes itself as a unique think/action tank that brings together all of the professional disciplines needed to study and combat substance abuse.

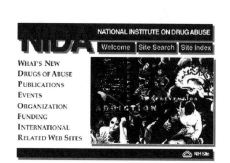

http://www.nida.nih.gov/
National Institute on Drug Abuse ★★
> Established in 1974, in 1992 becoming part of the National Institute of Health, this site contains links to research and papers to all areas of drugs and drug abuse. Invaluable resource.

http://www.ntis.gov/health/subabuse.htm
National Technical Information Service ★★
U.S. Department of Commerce
Springfield, Virginia
    Extensive information on substance abuse

http://www.drugs.indiana.edu/
On-line Dictionary of Street Drug Slang
    The Indiana Prevention Resource Center on-line dictionary
    contains nearly 1800 street drug slang terms.

http://PFPrevention.com/pfpmain.html
Physicians for Prevention ★
    Contains links to variety of resources physicians or other mental health workers can use in reviewing survey data; art with anti-substance abuse themes; screening instruments; links to local and national prevention organizations.

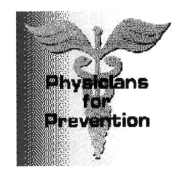

http://www.cts.com/crash/habtsmrt/hrmtitle.html
Push Harm Reduction ★
    Program designed by Robert Westermeyer, Harm Reduction is based on three central beliefs: (1) Excessive behaviors occur along a continuum of risk ranging from minimal to creative; (2) Changing addictive behavior is a stepwise process, complete abstinence being the final step; (3) Sobriety simply isn't for everybody.

http://www.netwizards.net/recovery/index.html
Recovery Online ★
    Links to all 12-Step programs; religious groups; secular groups; other recovery links.

http://members.aol.com/powerless/recovery.htm
Recovery Related Resources ★
    A collection of Internet sites put together to give a broad base of opinions, some of which are at variance with AA.

http://www.sad.org.uk/
Scotland Against Drugs ★
    An estimated 70 percent of thefts in Scotland are drug related. More than half of Scottish 16-year-old children have experimented with illegal drugs. This site contains local information for drug prevention and treatment.

http://www.winternet.com/%7Eterrym/sobriety.html
Sobriety and Recovery Resources ★★
    Lengthy listing of Internet resources dealing with all aspects of sobriety and addiction. Excellent resource.

http://peele.sas.nl/
Stanton Peele Addiction Web Site ★
    Stanton Peele presents a myriad of web sites dealing with most aspects of addiction. An alternative to the disease model.

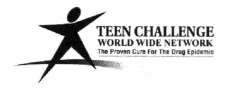

http://www.teenchallenge.com/
Teen Challenge: World Wide Network
> A non-profit organization dedicated to educating teens and adults about the dangers of drug abuse. Suggests there is hope and a new way of life for those already trapped or affected. Provides comprehensive facts and information about latest trends, statistics, slang, and signs associated with the drug culture.

http://www.mentalhealth.com/mag1/p5h-sb04.html
Treatment of Drug Abuse and Addiction
> Lengthy article from *Harvard Mental Health Letter.* Deals with all aspects of drug abuse and alcohol treatment.

http://www.wemac.com/safedrug.html
Unsafe and Safe Drugs for Recovering Addicts
> A partial list of medications and preparations considered to be unsafe for those recovering from the disease of chemical dependency (alcoholics and drug addicts).

Center for Substance Abuse Treatment

The Substance Abuse and Mental Health Services Administration
Department of Health and Human Services

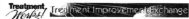

http://www.samhsa.gov/csat/csat.htm
U.S. Center for Substance Abuse Treatment ★
> Created in 1992 with the Congressional mandate to expand the availability of effective treatment and recovery services for alcohol and drug problems, CSAT works cooperatively across the private and public treatment spectrum to identify, develop, and support policies, approaches, and programs that enhance and expand treatment services to individuals who abuse alcohol and other drugs.

http://www.valleyhope.com/
The Valley Hope Association
Norton, Kansas
> Valley Hope operates treatment centers in Arizona, Colorado, Kansas, Missouri, Nebraska, and Oklahoma.

http://www.well.com/user/woa/
Web of Addictions ★★
> Dedicated to providing accurate information about drug and alcohol and other drug addictions. WOA is concerned about the pro-drug message in many web sites and use groups. Wants to provide a resource for teachers, students, and others who need factual information about abused drugs.

M. *Mailing Lists*

Acupuncture Treatment for Addiction and
   Mental Disorders
acudetox-1-request@lists.teleport.com
SUBSCRIBE ACUDETOX-L

Addiction Medicine
listserv@maelstrom.stjohns.edu
SUBSCRIBE ADD_MED

Canadian Society of Addiction Medicine
listserv@maelstrom.stjohns.edu
SUBSCRIBE CSAM

Addiction-Related Topics
listserv@listserv.kent.edu
SUBSCRIBE ADDICT-L

Breaking Free: Newsletter of the Addiction
   and Recovery Forum
listserv@listserv.aol.com
SUBSCRIBE BREAKING-FREE

Alcoholism Psychosocial Research Society
listserv@brownvm.brown.edu
SUBSCRIBE RSA-PS-L

Alcohol and Temperance History Group
listserv@miamiu.acs.muohio.edu
sub ATHG Your Name

Al-Anon/Alateen
listproc@solar.rtd.utk.edu
SUBSCRIBE AL-ANON Your Name

Controlled Drinking/Drug Use Discussion
listserv@maelstrom.stjohns.edu
SUBSCRIBE CD

Dual Diagnosis
listserv@sjuvm.stjohns.edu
SUBSCRIBE DUALDIAG Your Name

Jews in Recovery from Alcohol and Drugs
   (JACS)
listserv@sjuvm.stjohns.edu
SUBSCRIBE JACS Your Name

Journey to Recovery
listserv@maelstrom.stjohns.edu
SUBSCRIBE JOURNEY-TO-RECOVER

S.M.A.R.T. Recovery Self-Help List
listserv@maelstrom.stjohns.edu
SUBSCRIBE SMARTREC

No-smoke Quit Smoking
contact <angel2@qualcomm.com> or go to:
<http://www1.execnet.com/~joeym.ro.html>

Tobacco Talk
listserv@listserv.arizona.edu
sub TOBACTALK Your Name

SECTION V.
Schizophrenia and Other Psychotic Disorders

These disorders have psychotic symptoms as their defining feature. The following disorders are included:

A. Schizophrenia, a disturbance lasting at least 6 months and including two or more of the following: delusions, hallucinations, disorganized speech, grossly disorganized or catatonic behavior.

B. Schizophreniform Disorder, similar to schizophrenia except for duration, lasting from one to six months. A marked decline in functioning is not required.

C. Schizoaffective Disorder, a disturbance in which a mood episode and the active phase of schizophrenia occur together. Ordinarily preceded by two-week period of delusions or hallucinations.

D. Delusional Disorder, characterized by one month of nonbizarre delusions without other active-phase symptoms of schizophrenia.

E. Brief Psychotic Disorder (formerly Brief Reactive Psychosis), lasting from one day to one month.

F. Shared Psychotic Disorder (formerly Induced Psychotic Disorder), which develops in an individual influenced by someone else who has an established delusion with similar context.

A. *Schizophrenia*

http://www.appi.org/schizo.html
American Psychiatric Press Home Page ★
Contains hyperlinks to all aspects of schizophrenia.

http://www.mhsource.com/edu/psytimes/p950342.html
Childhood Schizophrenia
Good overview of childhood schizophrenia.

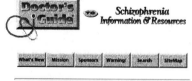

The latest medical news and information for patients or friends/parents of patients diagnosed with schizophrenia and schizophrenia-related disorders.

http://www.pslgroup.com/SCHIZOPHR.HTM
Doctor's Guide to Schizophrenia Information and Resources ★
References to medical news and alerts regarding schizophrenia. Contains many hyperlinks.

http://206.31.218.2/schiz/
HealthGuide: Schizophrenia ★
Discusses nature of schizophrenia, causes, symptoms, treatments, living with schizophrenia, working with healthcare professionals, organizations.

http://healthguide.com/schiz/
HealthGuide: Schizophrenia Can Be Inherited
Interesting information about schizophrenia.

 The Schizophrenia Homepage
www.schizophrenia.com

Living with Schizophrenia - The Email Newsletter -

http://www.schizophrenia.com/help/NewsL2.html
Living with Schizophrenia ★
A free newsletter via e-mail. Covers news regarding new treatments and medications; events for families, researchers and caregivers; updates on ongoing research; reviews of other websites.

http://www-personal.umich.edu/~jimmw
Meador-Woodruff Laboratory
Laboratory's primary research interest is understanding how different parts of the brain communicate with other parts via a variety of chemical signals, and how this communication is disrupted in schizophrenia.

http://pharminfo.com/pubs/msb/manschiz.html
Managing Schizophrenia
Brief article reprinted from the *Medical Sciences Bulletin*. Published by Pharmaceutical Information Associates, Ltd. Reviews some medications and their effectiveness.

http://www.ich.bpmf.ac.uk/units/mmschizo.htm
Molecular Medicine: Chromosome 22 and Schizophrenia
Technical article dealing with Chromosome 22 and Schizophrenia.

http://www/mhsource.com/narsad.html
National Alliance for Research on Schizophrenia and Depression ★
Great Neck, New York
Contains many hyperlinks including NARSAD FAQ, OCD symptoms in schizophrenia, link between nicotine and schizophrenia. Also available in Spanish.

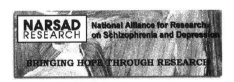

http://www.nsf.org.uk/
National Schizophrenia Fellowship
U. K.
A national voluntary organization which campaigns on behalf of, and provides support to, people with a severe mental illness, particularly schizophrenia, their families and caregivers. Has 8 centers in the U.K.

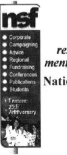

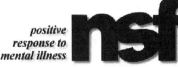

positive response to mental illness
National Schizophrenia Fellowship

NSF exists to improve the lives of everyone affected by severe mental illnesses by providing quality support, services and information and by influencing local, regional and national policies.

http://www.mhsource.com/edu/psytimes/p960121.html
Prenatal Risk Factors in Schizophrenia
> Review of prenatal exposures with emphasis on prenatal infection, prenatal nutritional deficiency, and obstetric complications.

http://www.psychiatry.uq.edu.au/qcsr/qcsr.htm
Queensland Centre for Schizophrenia Research ★
Brisbane, Australia
> Established with the aim of studying schizophrenia utilizing a multidisciplinary approach. Emphasis is on research for improving knowledge and treatment.

http://www.mentalhealth.com/dis-rs3/p26-ps01.html
Research regarding Cause ★
> Extensive pages detailing hundreds of studies on the cause of schizophrenia.

http://www.mentalhealth.com/dis-rsl/p24-ps01.html
Research regarding Diagnosis ★
> Extensive pages detailing research studies regarding the diagnosis of schizophrenia.

http://www.noah.cuny.edu/illness/mentalhealth/cornell/resources/schizore.html
Resources: Schizophrenia
> Books and organizations dealing with schizophrenia.

http://www.mentalhealth.com/book/p40-sc01.html
Schizophrenia: A Handbook For Families ★
> Published by Health Canada in cooperation with the Schizophrenia Society of Canada, the *Handbook* is an extremely valuable resource guide covering every aspect of this disorder. Contains many hyperlinks.

http://www.mentalhealth.com/dis1/p21-ps01.html
Schizophrenia: American Description
> Gives diagnostic criteria, schizophrenia subtypes (paranoid, catatonic, disorganized, undifferentiated, residual), associated features, differential diagnosis.

| Schizophrenia and Mental Health Resources of Interest on the Internet |

http://www.yale.edu/vayale/internet.html
Schizophrenia and Mental Health: Resources on the Internet ★★
VA-Yale University
> List of internet resources referring to all aspects of schizophrenia and mental health.

http://www.mentalhealth.com/book/p42-sc5.html
Schizophrenia: Course and Outcome ★
> Contains questions regarding meaning of the diagnosis, common misconceptions about course and outcome, how to improve chances, what relatives can do. Useful hyperlinks.

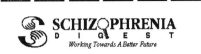

http://www.vaxxine.com/schizophrenia/
Schizophrenia Digest ★
> Contains helpful hints, personal profiles, as well as articles on treatments, medications, and new developments.

http://www.schizophrenia.com/
Schizophrenia Home Page ★
> Attempts to be the leading non-profit web resource and education center for schizophrenia. Offers current news and events, online support and discussion groups, information for families and friends, information for people who have schizophrenia, information for researchers and professionals, information for students. Many hyperlinks.

http://www.aacap.org/web/aacap/factsfam/schizo.htm
Schizophrenia in Children
> From American Academy of Child and Adolescent Psychiatry, lists early warning signs.

http://mentalhealth.com/book/p42-sc1.html
Schizophrenia: Returning Home
> Excellent information regarding what happens after discharge, coping at home, need for extra help, booklets for reference.

http://www.schizophrenia.ca/
Schizophrenia Society of Canada ★
Toronto, Canada
> Discusses nature of schizophrenia, various provincial associations, links to many other sites. English and French.

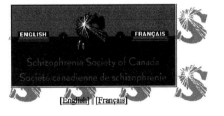

http://www.mentalhealth.com/book/p40-sc04.html
Schizophrenia: Questions and Answers ★
> By David Shore, National Institute of Mental Health. Contains information on nature of schizophrenia, causes, treatment, how other people can help, outlook, how to subscribe to *Schizophrenia Bulletin*.

http://members.aol.com/leonardjk/support.htm
Schizophrenia Support Organizations ★
> A listing of support organizations for people with Schizophrenia and their families. Contains hyperlinks to organizations in Australia, Bermuda, Canada, England, India, Ireland, New Zealand, and the USA.

http://www.mhsource.com/edu/psytimes/p950627.html
Treatment of Schizophrenics: Trends and Outlook
> Offers good overview of developments and the therapeutic effects of medications.

http://www.mentalhealth.com/book/p40-sc02.html
Youth's Greatest Disabler ★
British Columbia, Canada

> Contains very lengthy information for young people, educators, parents and others. Discusses various aspects of schizophrenia: no one is immune, what schizophrenia really is, what causes schizophrenia, symptoms, early warning signs, types of schizophrenia, what it is like to have schizophrenia, how schizophrenia affects families, the "blame and shame" syndrome, the role of families, getting treatment, promising developments, medication update, recovery, FAQ, education and schizophrenia, stigma and discrimination, effect of stigma on research, research funding, schizophrenia and violence, British Columbia Schizophrenia Society and branches, resource materials, glossary.

B. *Schizophreniform Disorder*

<u>Schizophreniform Disorder</u>

Research

http://mentalhealth.com/dis-rs1/p24-ps04.html
Schizophreniform Disorder: Research

> Summary of research articles.

C. *Schizoaffective Disorder*

http://www.noah.cuny.edu/illness/mentalhealth/cornell/conditions/schizoaf.html
Fact Sheet: Schizoaffective Disorder ★

> From New York Hospital, Cornell Medical Center, Ask Noah Series. Presents a fact sheet dealing with definition, symptoms, cause, course, treatment, self-management, dealing with relapse, further information and support.

http://www.mentalhealth.com/mag1/p5h-scf2.html
Schizoaffective Disorder

> Discussion of symptoms, causes, and treatment.

http://www.mentalhealth.com/dis1/p21-ps05.html
Schizoaffective Disorder: American Description

> Detailed criteria for schizoaffective disorder.

http://mentalhealth.com/dis-rs1/p24-ps04.html
Schizoaffective Disorder: Cause

> Summary of research articles regarding cause of schizoaffective disorder.

http://www.mentalhealth.com/rx/p23-ps05.html
Schizoaffective Disorder: Treatment

> Medical and psychosocial treatments.

D. *Delusional Disorder*

http://www.mentalhealth.com/dis1/p21-ps02.html
Diagnostic Criteria: American Description
    Detailed criteria for diagnosis of delusional disorder.

http://www.mentalhealth.com/dis-rs3/p26-ps02.html
Research regarding Cause
    Summary of research articles regarding cause of delusional disorder.

http://www.mentalhealth.com/dis-rs1/p24-ps02.html
Research regarding Diagnosis
    Summary of research articles regarding diagnosis of delusional disorder.

http://www.mentalhealth.com/rx/p23-ps02.html
Treatment
    Medical and psychosocial treatment modalities.

E. *Brief Psychotic Disorder (formerly Brief Reactive Psychosis)*

http://mentalhealth.com/dis-rs1/p24-ps03.html
Research
    Summary of research articles regarding brief psychotic disorder.

F. *Shared Psychotic Disorder (formerly Induced Psychotic Disorder)*

http://www.mentalhealth.com/dis1/p21-ps06.html
American Description
    Diagnostic criteria, associated features, and differential diagnosis.

http://www.mentalhealth.com/dis-rs1/p24-ps06.html
Research
    Summary of research articles regarding shared psychotic disorder.

G. *Miscellaneous Internet Site*

http://home.vicnet.net.au/~eppic
Early Psychosis Prevention and Intervention ★
Victoria, Australia

> A program from the Center for Young People's Mental Health,
> Western Health Care Network, which offers an integrated and
> comprehensive psychiatric service aimed at addressing the
> needs of older adolescents and young adults with emerging
> psychotic disorders in Melbourne. The program has been
> developed in response to perceived flaws in the way young
> people with psychotic disorder have been traditionally treated.
> Many hyperlinks.

M. *Mailing Lists*

Madness
listserv@sjuvm.stjohns.edu
SUB Madness Your Name

Schizophrenia
http://www.mhsource.com/interactive/mailinglist.html
Use subscription form

Schizophrenia Discussion Group
listserv@maelstrom.stjohns.edu
SUBSCRIBE SCHIZOPH

MHI Schizophrenia Discussion
majordomo@mhsource.com
Use subscription form

Mood Disorders

Mood disorders are divided into two main categories:

A. Depressive Disorders
- i. Major Depressive Disorder. A period of at least 2 weeks during which there is either depressed mood or the loss of interest or pleasure in nearly all activities.
- ii. Dysthymic Disorder. Depressed mood for most of the day, for more days than not, as indicated by either subjective account or observation by others, for at least 2 years.

B. Bipolar Disorder
- i. Bipolar Disorder I. Presence of only one manic episode and no past major depressive episodes.
- ii. Bipolar Disorder II. Presence of one or more major depressive episodes, history of at least one hypomanic episode and a condition in which there has never been a manic episode or a mixed episode.
- iii. Cyclothymic Disorder. A condition lasting at least 2 years with the presence of numerous periods of hypomanic symptoms and numerous periods of depressive symptoms that do not meet the criteria for major depressive episode.

C. Miscellaneous Mood Disorders
- i. Postpartum Depression. Severe depression with an onset within 4 weeks after delivery of a child.
- ii. Seasonal Affective Disorder. Severe depression at characteristic times of the year. Usually begins in fall or winter and remits in spring.
- iii. Suicide. Taking of one's own life.

A. *Depressive Disorders*

i. MAJOR DEPRESSIVE DISORDERS

http://www.mentalhealth.com/mag1/p51-dp01.html
Adolescent Depression
Excellent discussion by Maurice Blackman, University of Alberta Hospitals, Edmonton, concerning adolescent depression.

http://www.blarg.com/~charlatn/Depression.html
Andrew's Depression Page ★
Compiled by Andrew Fineberg, contains important documents concerning depression: FAQ; voices of depression; treatment; children; suicide; mental health; resources; mood scales; etc.

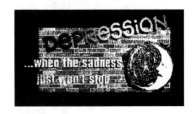

http://www.mediconsult.com/depression/drugs/content.html
Depression Drug Information
> A listing of brand and generic names as well as the general category. A keyword search field for any unlisted drug.

http://www.cmhc.com/perspectives/articles/art11967.htm
Depression in Brain Injury
> Daniel Gardner discusses the need for a comprehensive.biological/psychological/social approach to evaluation and treatment of depression in brain injury cases.

http://www.fis.utoronto.ca/~gruppuso/depress.htm
Depression on the Internet ★★
University of Toronto
> Mary Ann Gruppuso offers links to articles discussing the nature of depression; how one finds information on the Internet; resources; bibliography.

DEPRESSION QUESTIONNAIRE 2

Goldbery Depression Inventory
Ivan Goldberg

Use this questionnaire to help determine if you need to see a mental health professional for diagnosis and treatment of depression.

http://www.cmhc.com/guide/dep2quiz.htm
Depression Questionnaire
> The Goldberg Depression Inventory designed for a non- professional to determine whether there is need to see a mental health professional for further diagnosis and treatment of depression.

http://earth.execpc.com/~corbeau
Depression Resources List ★
> Good compilation of hyperlinks to resources dealing with depression, bipolar disorder, panic and suicide.

http://pharminfo.com/drugfaq/antidep_faq.html
DrugFAQ's: Antidepressants
> Discusses specific antidepressants and FAQ from the University of Maryland Drug Information Service.

http://kendaco.telebyte.com/~cgrandy/shoc_idx.html
Electro-Shock or Electro-Convulsive Therapy
> A clearing house for information on the dangers of ECT.

http://www.cmhc.com/guide/ect.htm
Electroconvulsive Therapy ★
> Excellent resource on ECT treatment for depression..Discusses anesthetic considerations, biased media reports, Johns Hopkins program, and a statement from National Alliance for the Mentally Ill regarding the advantages of ECT.

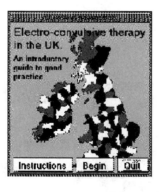

http://www.ambrosia.demon.co.uk/psych/ect.htm
Electroconvulsive Therapy ★
> An introduction to ECT suitable for medical and nursing staff new to psychiatry, but also of interest to other people. Good links.

http://www-leland.stanford.edu/~yesavage/GDS.html
Geriatric Depression Scale
>   Information on a basic screening measure for depression in older adults.

http://healthguide.com/dep/
HealthGuide: Depression ★
>   Discusses incidence of depression, general listing of symptoms, causes of depression, types of depression, medications, psychotherapy, resources.

http://healthguide.com/Pharmacy/ssris.htm
HealthGuide Pharmacy—SSRI's
>   Discusses SSRIs as newer antidepressants that treat the symptoms of depression more effectively than TCAs and often produce less troublesome side effects.

http://www.mentalhealth.com/dx/dx-md01.html
Major Depressive Disorder: Online Diagnosis
>   An evaluation for patients as an initial screening in preparation for a diagnosis by a mental health professional.

http://www.cmhc.com/disorders/sx5.htm
Major Depressive Episode: Symptoms
>   Presents criteria for diagnosing a major depressive episode not seen as a disorder in itself, but as a part of another disorder.

http://www.mentalhealth.com/rx/p23-md01.html
Major Depressive Disorder: Treatment ★
>   Excellent and lengthy resource which discusses psychotherapy vs. pharmacotherapy, psychosocial therapies, medical therapies and medications. Offers references with many hyperlinks.

http://depression.org/
National Foundation for Depressive Illness ★
New York, New York
>   The Foundation offers hyperlinks and references regarding the consequences of depression, symptoms, what can be done, severe depression as a biochemical illness, and other very useful information.

http://www.med.nyu.edu/Psych/screens/depres.html
Online Depression Screening Test
>   Brief screening for depression from NYU Department of Psychiatry.

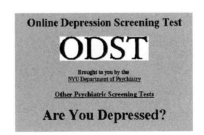

http://members.aol.com/drjnh/pdt.htm
Personalized Depression Therapy: A New Treatment
>   A therapy based on premise that depression is a behavioral response and can be reprogrammed. Presents information on how to.purchase a videotape and manual and to access unlimited e-mail support.

http://www.healthtouch.com/level/leaflets/nimh/nimh015.htm
Ten Ways to Help a Depressed Person
Ten common sense pieces of advice.

http://www.odos.uiuc.edu/Counseling_Center/depress.htm
Understanding Depression
Discusses depression in general and presents symptoms of.depression, indicating the negative effects on a person's life.

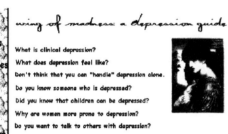

http://members.aol.com/depress/index.htm
Wing of Madness: A Depression Guide ★
Definition, diagnosis, and treatment of depression; resources for clinical depression and related illnesses; personal.experiences; special groups and situations; FAQ; medications.

http://none.coolware.com/health/medical_reporter/depress.html
Women and Depression
Explains how to obtain brochure "Depression: What Every Woman Should Know," available from the National Institute of Mental Health's Depression Awareness, Recognition and Treatment Program.

ii. DYSTHYMIC DISORDERS

http://www.mentalhealth.com/dis1/p21-md04.html
Dysthymia: American Description
Presents diagnostic criteria and associated features for dysthymic disorder.

http://www.mentalhealth.com/dis-rs3/p26-md04.html
Dysthymia: Research regarding Cause
Summaries of research articles dealing with the causes of dysthymic disorder.

http://www.mentalhealth.com/dis-rs1/p24-md04.html
Dysthymia: Research regarding Diagnosis
Very lengthy summaries of research articles dealing with the diagnosis of dysthymic disorder.

http://www.mentalhealth.com/dis-rs2/p25-md04.html
Dysthymia: Research regarding Treatment
Lengthy summaries of research articles dealing with treatment of dysthymic disorder.

Dysthymic Disorder

Treatment

http://www.mentalhealth.com/rx/p23-md04.html
Dysthymic Disorder: Treatment
Discusses dysthymic disorder treatment from the medical and psychosocial viewpoints.

B. *Bipolar Disorders*

i. BIPOLAR I AND II

http://www.pendulum.org
Pendulum Resources ★
> Deals specifically with bipolar disorder.

http://www.frii.com/%7Eparrot/bip.html
Bipolar Disorder ★
> Diagnostic criteria; additional definitions; personal experiences; available treatments; suicide and bipolar disorder; learning about your own diagnosis; special resources; files and web links.

http://www.moodswing.org/
Bipolar Information Network ★
> An information source for bipolar and mood disorders. References books, a bipolar forum, supports, links, etc.

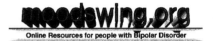

http://healthguide.com/Bipolar
Health Guide: Bipolar Disorder ★
> Excellent hyperlinks dealing with definitions, symptoms,. related disorders, medical treatments, therapy, hospital stay, and resources.

http://www.sstar.com/jsharai/index.htm
Heart Speaketh to Heart
> Discusses the link between alcoholism and manic depression.

http://www.deancare.com/info/info16.htm
Lithium Information Center ★
> The Dean Foundation for Health, Research and Education, Madison, Wisconsin
> More than 27,000 references on all aspects of lithium.

http://www.psych.med.umich.edu/web/aacap/factsFam/bipolar.htm
Manic-Depressive Illness in Teens
> Reviews manic and depressive symptoms and how these can manifest in adolescence.

http://www.mentalhealth.com/sw/p71-mood.html
Mood Disorder Diagnostic Program
> A computerized diagnostic program available to therapists or patients. Offers diagnosis for bipolar disorder, cyclothymia, major depression, dysthymia, and organic mood disorder.

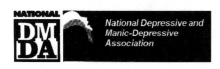

http://www.ndmda.org/
National Depressive and Manic-Depressive Association ★
Chicago, Illinois

> Excellent resource discussing all aspect of depressive and manic-depressive disorders. Offers information regarding advocacy, suicide, success stories, ask a doc, etc.

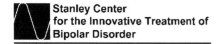

http://www.wpic.pitt.edu/STANLEY/
Stanley Center for the Innovative Treatment of Bipolar Disorder ★
Pittsburgh, Pennsylvania

> Includes the bipolar registry, clinical trials, and the provider consortium. Potential registrants from the U.S. and Canada may call (800) 424-7657.

ii. CYCLOTHYMIC DISORDERS

http://www.mentalhealth.com/dis1/p21-md03.html
Cyclothymic Disorder: American Description

> Diagnostic criteria, associated features, differential diagnosis.

http://www.mentalhealth.com/dis-rsl/p24-md03.html
Cyclothymic Disorder: Research

> A summary of research studies.

http://www.mentalhealth.com/rx/p23-md03.html
Cyclothymic Disorder: Treatment

> Medical treatments and psychosocial treatments.

C. *Miscellaneous Mood Disorders*

i. POSTPARTUM DEPRESSION

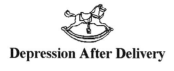

Depression After Delivery

http://www.behavenet.com/dadinc/#DAD
Depression after Delivery ★

> Reviews causes, treatments, symptoms, depression and psychosis. Many resources.

http://siteguider.com/postpart.htm
Postpartum: After the Baby

> Practical advice with many hyperlinks to concerns over postpartum care, adjustment, birth control, thyroid dysfunction, etc.

http://www.mhsource.com/edu/psytimes/p961028.html
Postpartum Mood Disorders ★

> Presents the symptomatology of "baby blues" as compared to postpartum depression; offers scientific research on hormonal and other biological factors; discusses pharmacologic, electroconvulsive, and self-help approaches to treatment.

http://users.penn.com/~dgenung/ppd.html
Web Page Index on Postpartum Depression ★
> Reviews symptoms of PPD. Contains many PPD Support. Links.

ii. SEASONAL AFFECTIVE DISORDER

http://www.outsidein.co.uk/bodyclock/sadinfo.htm
S.A.D.: Outside Information ★
Describes SAD, from Outside In, U.K.

http://www.psych.helsinki.fi/~janne/mood/sad.html
Winter Depression: S.A.D. Information
Basic information from Mary Jacobs.

**Winter Depression
(Seasonal Affective Disorder, SAD)
Information**

iii. SUICIDE

http://www.cyberpsych.org/aas.htm
American Association of Suicidology ★
Washington, D.C.
> An educational resource discussing membership information, suicide prevention guidelines from the Center for Disease Control and Prevention, case worker exam information, suicide prevention papers.

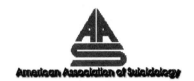

http://www.afsp.org/
American Foundation for Suicide Prevention ★
New York, New York
> Produced by a grant from Solvay Pharmaceuticals, this site presents suicide facts, articles regarding depression and suicide, research articles, suicide support, suicide and AIDS, and information about the AFSP program.

http://www.virtualcity.com/youthsuicide/
Gay and Bisexual Male Youth Suicidality Studies ★
> Studies shedding light on male youth suicide problems and related negative issues in research and mental health.

http://www.yellowribbon.org/
Light for Life: Prevention of Youth Suicide ★
> Program for the prevention of youth suicide called Yellow Ribbon Program. Intended for teens and youth so that they have a.resource to contact when in a crisis.

http://www.save.org/
SAVE: Educating about Suicide ★
> Many hyperlinks dealing with untreated depression as the #1 cause of suicide.

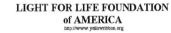

**LIGHT FOR LIFE FOUNDATION
of AMERICA**
http://www.yellowribbon.org
Our mission is to save lives through the use of the Yellow Ribbon Program to eliminate youth suicide.

Suicide kills our children *3 to 6 times more than homicide.* There are 16 teen suicides a day in the United States. Because of the internal nature of depression and loneliness, thousands of our children who appear to be happy are screaming silently in the deepest emotional pain, what can we do?

We can reach out to youth and help them with the Yellow Ribbon Card program! The card is a business sized card that teen and youth can keep with them so they may use it to ask for help when they are at a time of crisis.

http://www.lib.ox.ac.uk/internet/news/faq/archive/suicide
.info.html
Suicide: Frequently Asked Questions ★
> Attempts to raise awareness about suicide to help people in crisis, showing how to seek help and make better choices. Lengthy and informative.

http://www.siec.ca/
Suicide Information and Education ★
> Contains information regarding Resources, SIED library, FAQ, training programs, helpful organizations, and crisis centers.

SPAN
SUICIDE PREVENTION ADVOCACY NETWORK
ADVOCATES DEVELOPMENT OF A PROVEN,
EFFECTIVE SUICIDE PREVENTION PROGRAM

http://www.spanusa.org/
Suicide Prevention Advocacy Program
Marietta, Georgia
> Q and A regarding Suicide Prevention Advocacy Network (SPAN); letters to Congress; info re National Awareness Day.

http://www.rochford.org/suicide/
The Real World: Suicide ★
> Information about suicide and its prevention, including FAQ, statistics, international crisis resources, and links to other suicide sites.

D. *Miscellaneous Internet Sites for Depression*

http://www.execpc.com/~corbeau/best.html
Best Things to Say to Someone Who Is Depressed
> Excellent responses.

Welcome to
Dr. Ivan's DEPRESSION CENTRAL

This site is Internet's central clearing house for information on all types of depressive disorders and on the most effective treatments for individuals suffering from Major Depression, Manic-Depression (Bipolar Disorder), Cyclothymia, Dysthymia and other mood disorders.

---

http://psycom.net/depression.central.html
Dr. Ivan's Depression Central
> A clearinghouse for information on all types of depressive disorders and the most effective treatments for individuals suffering from major depression, manic-depression (bipolar disorder), cyclothymia, dysthymia, and other mood disorders.

http://www.span.com.au/moodswing/index/html
Mood Disorders Association
Marleston, South Australia
> Non-profit, non-denominational association formed in Adelaide in 1983. Primary aim is to provide active support for sufferers of moodswings and their families.

http://www.execpc.com/~corbeau/worst.html
Worst Things to Say to Someone Who Is Depressed
Excellent responses.

E. *Mailing Lists*

Bipolar
http://www.mhsource.com/mailinglist.html
use subscription form

Bipolar
majordomo@Esosoft.com
SUBSCRIBE ROSEANDTHORNS

Bipolar
majordomo@ncar.ucar.edu
SUBSCRIBE PENDULUM Your e-mail address

Depression
http://www.mhsource.com/interactive/mail-
inglist.html
use subscription form

Depression
majordomo@world.std.com
SUBSCRIBE WALKERS

Depression
listserv@soundprint.brandywine.american.edu
SUBSCRIBE DEPRESS

Depression, Christian Oriented
hub@xc.org
SUBSCRIBE XN-DEPRESSION

Depression and Emotional Trauma
majordomo@userhome.com
SUBSCRIBE SYBIL

Suicide Support
majordomo@research.canon.com.au
SUB SUICIDE-SUPPORT Your Name

Anxiety Disorders

The *DSM-IV* lists the following disorders:

A. Panic attacks, characterized by sudden onset of intense apprehension, fearfulness or terror, often with a sense of impending doom. Physiological symptoms often reported.
B. Agoraphobia, characterized by anxiety about or avoidance of situations from which escape might be difficult.
C. Phobias, characterized by irrational fears.
D. Obsessive-Compulsive Disorder, characterized by obsessions or compulsions.
E. Posttraumatic Stress Disorder, characterized by the reexperiencing of a traumatic event often accompanied by physiological symptoms.
F. Anxiety, characterized by excessive worry.

A. *Panic Attacks*

Welcome to the Anxiety Panic internet resource, **a grass roots project involving thousands of people interested in anxiety disorders such as panic attacks, phobias, shyness, generalized anxiety, obsessive-compulsive behavior and post traumatic stress. tAPir is a self-help network dedicated to the overcoming and cure of overwhelming anxiety.**

http://www.algy.com/anxiety/menu.shtml
Anxiety-Panic Internet Resource ★★
> A grass-roots project involving thousands of people interested in anxiety disorders, such as panic attacks, phobias, shyness, generalized anxiety, obsessive-compulsive disorder, and posttraumatic stress. A self-help network dedicated to overcoming and curing overwhelming anxiety.

http://www.nimh.nih.gov/publicat/gettreat.htm
Getting Treated for Panic Disorder ★
> To determine whether one has a panic disorder and how it can be effectively treated.

http://www.mentalheatlh.com/mag1/p5h-pan3.html
Panic and Suicide
> Brief exerpt from a study by NIMH revealing that people who suffer from panic disorder are at much greater risk of suicide than previously suspected.

http://www.mentalhealth.com/dis1/p21-an01.html
Panic Disorder: American Description
> Diagnostic criteria for panic disorder.

http://www.mentalhealth.com/dis-rsl/p24-an01.html
Panic Disorder: Diagnosis
> Diagnostic criteria. Discusses criteria for panic disorder with
> and without agoraphobia. Lists associated features and differ-
> ential diagnoses.

http://www.mentalhealth.com/rx/p23-an01.html
Panic Disorder: Treatment
> Reviews medical and psychosocial treatments.

http://www.nimh.nih.gov/publicat/pandtr.htm
Panic Disorder: Treatment and Referral
> Information for health care professionals. Discusses panic dis-
> order, causes, who can treat, how the professional can talk to
> the patient, sources for further information.

http://e2.empirenet.com/~berta/
Treat Your Own Panic Disorder ★
> Reviews self-treatment for panic disorder. A self-help approach
> including chapters on how to succeed, panic and hyperventila-
> tion, breathing in and out, daily practice in breathing,
> advanced exercises.

http://text.nlm.nih.gov/nih/cdc/www/85txt.html
Treatment of Panic Disorder ★
> Lengthy and comprehensive article from National Institutes of
> Health Consensus Development Conference in September 1991.

B. *Agoraphobia*

http://www.mentalhealth.com/dx/dx-an02.html
Agoraphobia: Diagnosis
> Brief description of criteria for agoraphobia. Offers online test
> to assist in psychiatric diagnosis.

http://www.mentalhealth.com/dis1/p21-an02.html
**Agoraphobia Without History of Panic Disorder: American
Description**
> Diagnostic criteria and associated features.

http://www.mentalhealth.com/dis-rs3/p26-an02.html
**Agoraphobia Without History of Panic Disorder: Research Re
Cause**
> A brief summary of two research studies.

http://www.mentalhealth.com/dis-rs1/p24-an02.html
Agoraphobia Without History of Panic Disorder: Diagnosis
> Summary of many research articles.

> HOW TO TREAT YOUR OWN
> PANIC DISORDER

http://www.mentalhealth.com/dis-rs2/p25-an02.html
Agoraphobia Without History of Panic Disorder: Treatment
Summary of research articles.

http://ijvr.uccs.edu/north.htm
Treatment of Agoraphobia
A study that investigated the effectiveness of a virtual environment desensitization in the treatment of agoraphobia. The virtual environment desensitization was shown to be effective.

C. *Phobias*

The Phobia List

http://www.sonic.net/~fredd/phobia1.html
Phobia List ★
Compiled by Fred Culbertson. Interesting and comprehensive
listing of every known phobia and its definition. Excellent for
trivia games!

http://www.mentalhealth.com/dis1/p21-an04.html
Specific Phobia: American Description
Diagnostic criteria for specific phobia (formerly known as sim-
ple phobia).

http://www.mentalhealth.com/dx/dx-an04.html
Specific Phobia: Diagnosis
Brief description of criteria to diagnose agoraphobia. Online
test to aid in psychiatric diagnosis.

http://www.mentalhealth.com/dis-rs1/p24-an04.html
Specific Phobia: Research
Summary of research studies dealing with specific phobia (for-
merly known as simple phobia).

http://www.mentalhealth.com/rx/p23-an04.html
Specific Phobia: Treatment
Medical and psychosocial treatments for specific phobia.

D. *Obsessive-Compulsive Disorder*

http://members.aol.com/cherlene/ocd.html
Cherry's Website: OCD Caterpillars into Butterflies ★
Cherry writes a book about people and their experiences with
OCD. Goal is to give hope to others with OCD, to help people
help themselves, and to assist families in helping their loved ones.

**Back to
HealthGuide
Online!**   **Obsessive-Compulsive
Disorder**

http://206.31.218.2/ocd/
Health Guide: OCD ★
Discusses OCD, how to live with this condition, whom it
affects, causes, treatment, resources.

http://members.aol.com/west24th/index.html
Obsessive Compulsive Anonymous ★

A fellowship of people who share experience, strength, and hope with each other to solve common problems and to help others recover from OCD. No dues or fees. Contains information regarding tools for recovery, phone calls and writing, prayers and meditation, anonymity, abstinence, slogans, hyperlinks to meetings and resources.

http://www.mentalhealth.com/dis1/p21-an05.html
Obsessive Compulsive Disorder: American Description

Diagnostic criteria for obsessive-compulsive disorder.

http://fairlite.com/ocd
Obsessive Compulsive Disorder: Bulletin Board ★

Sponsored by Fairlite Counseling Center. Contains many hyperlinks to information regarding medications, *DSM-IV* definitions, medical resources, personal resources, bulletin board, etc.

http://www.nimh.nih.gov/publicat/ocd.htm
Obsessive Compulsive Disorder ★

From the NIMH. Discusses OCD, frequency, key features, causes, treatment, getting help, family issues, special needs, further information, and references.

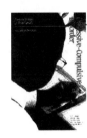

Obsessive-Compulsive Disorder

What is OCD?
How common is OCD?
Key Features of OCD
What causes OCD?
Do I have OCD?
Treatment of OCD; Progress Through Research
How to Get Help for OCD
What the Family Can Do to Help
Continuing Research
If You Have Special Needs
For Further Information
References

http://www.mentalheatlh.com/dis-rs1/p24-an05.html
Obsessive Compulsive Disorder: Research regarding Diagnosis

Lengthy summary of research articles dealing with OCD.

http://pages.prodigy.com/alwillen/ocf.html
Obsessive Compulsive Foundation ★
Milford, Connecticut

Offers comprehensive sites regarding OCD. Good hyperlinks.

http://www.mentalhealth.com/dis-rs3/p26-an05.html
Obsessive Compulsive Disorder: Research regarding Cause

Lengthy summary of research articles dealing with the causes of OCD.

http://www.mentalhealth.com/dis-rs1/p24-an05.html
Obsessive Compulsive Disorder: Research regarding Diagnosis

Lengthy summary of research articles dealing with OCD.

http://www.mentalhealth.com//dis-rs2/p25-an05.html
Obsessive Compulsive Disorder: Research regarding Treatment

Lengthy summary of research articles dealing with treatment of OCD.

http://www.mentalhealth.com//mag1/p5h-ocd5.html
Obsessive Compulsive Disorder: Comparison of Treatments
> Edna Foa, Center for Treatment and Study of Anxiety, Medical College of Pennsylvania, discusses behavior therapy effectiveness compared to medication.

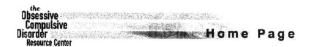

http://www.ocdresource.com/
OCD Resource Center ★
> Provided by Pharmacia & Upjohn and Solvay Pharmaceuticals. Information is offered regarding all aspects of OCD, emphasizing pharmacological treatment.

http://www.mentalhealth.com/dis-rs2/p25-an05.html
Obsessive Compulsive Disorder: Treatment ★
> Lengthy summary of research articles dealing with the treatment of OCD.

E. *Posttraumatic Stress Disorder*

http://trauma-pages.com/
Baldwin's Trauma Information Pages ★★
> Provides information about traumatic stress for clinicians and researchers in the field. Baldwin's interests include both clinical and research aspects of trauma responses and their resolution.

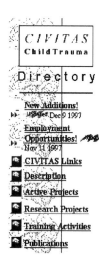

http://www.bcm.tmc.edu/civitas/description.html
Civitas Child Trauma Programs Home Page
> From the Baylor College of Medicine. Provides useful information and educational materials.

http://gladstone.uoregon.edu/~dvb/goodwin.htm
Etiology of Combat-Related Posttraumatic Stress Disorders ★
> Jim Goodwin writes prolifically about this disorder and its etiology. Required reading for all professionals working with this population.

http://www.jimhopper.com/
Hopper's Home Page ★
> Pre-doc psychology intern Hopper's graduate research focuses on the effects of child abuse, especially on men. Contains many pages dealing with the impact of early abuse on males. Even as a student, Jim Hopper is contributing much to this field! Good hyperlinks.

http://www.bcm.tmc.edu/civitas/publicat/incubated1.html
Incubated in Terror: Neurodevelopmental Factors in Cycle of Violence
> Comprehensive article by Bruce Perry from Baylor College of Medicine.

http://www.mcs.net/~kathyw/trauma.html
Information on Trauma and Dissociation ★
> A series of resources for all aspects of trauma and dissociation.

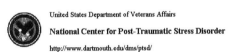
↑Essential Information on Trauma and Dissociation

http://www.istss.com
International Society for Traumatic Stress Studies
Northbrook, Illinois
> Founded in 1985, ISTSS provides a forum for sharing research, clinical strategies, public policy, concerns, and theoretical formulation of trauma in the U.S. and around the world.

http://www.xs4all.nl/~mtrapman/
Mental Health for Children and Youth in Armed Conflict
> Marc-Jan Trapman's Home Page presents documents prepared for a Conference on Trauma of Children and Youth presented at the The Hague in November 1995.

http://www.dartmouth.edu/dms/ptsd/About.html
Literature on PTSD ★
> A bibliographical database, sponsored by U.S. Department of Veterans Affairs, PILOTS (Published International Literature On Traumatic Stress) offers references for literature dealing with PTSD and other mental health sequelae of traumatic events, without disciplinary, linguistic, or geographical limitations and presenting both current and retrospective coverage. Valuable despite stilted language!

United States Department of Veterans Affairs

National Center for Post-Traumatic Stress Disorder

http://www.dartmouth.edu/dms/ptsd/

About the PILOTS Database

PILOTS is a bibliographical database covering Published International Literature On Traumatic Stress. It is produced at the headquarters of the National Center for Post-Traumatic Stress Disorder in White River Junction, Vermont. Although it is sponsored by the U.S. Department of Veterans Affairs, the PILOTS database is not limited to literature on PTSD among veterans. Its goal is to include citations to all literature on PTSD and other mental-health sequelae of traumatic events, without disciplinary, linguistic, or geographical limitations, and to offer both current and retrospective coverage.

http://www.clinicalsocialwork.com/
McClendon's Clinical Social Work Home Page ★★
> Pat McClendon writes about all types of trauma on the minds and bodies of survivors. Identifies and communicates effective treatment protocols for trauma survivors. Good resource!

http://uhs.bsd.uchicago.edu/~bhsiung/tips/ptsd.html
Medications for Combat PTSD ★
> Jonathan Shay from the Boston VA Outpatient Clinic presents a listing of medications. Prepared as educational material for combat veterans, it is also useful for spouses as well as nonphysician mental health professionals. Many hyperlinks.

U.S. Department of Veterans Affairs
National Center for PTSD
Research and Education on
Post-Traumatic Stress Disorder

http://www.dartmouth.edu/dms/ptsd/
National Center for PTSD ★
White River, Vermont

Maintained by the U. S. Department of Veterans Affairs, National Center for PTSD, the Center carries out a broad range of multidisciplinary activities in research, education, and training. Discusses the Center and offers hyperlinks to seven divisional consortium branches. Hyperlinks to the PILOTS database; selected publications; positions available; links to other WWW sites. Also links to information for veterans, students, therapists, researchers and trauma survivors.

http://www.dartmouth.edu/dms/ptsd/Clinicians.html
Post Traumatic Diagnosis and Treatment

Written for mental health clinicians by Matthew Friedman, Dartmouth Medical School. Focuses on four issues: PTSD assessment; treatment approaches; therapist issues; and current controversies.

http://www.mentalhealth.com/dis1/p21-an06.html
PTSD: American Description

Diagnostic criteria for PTSD.

Post-Traumatic Stress Disorder Bibliography

An annotated list of books and articles about the emotional aftershocks of rape, incest, child abuse, street crime, family violence, war, Holocaust, racial violence, political terror, and other forms of psychological trauma.

---

http://www.sover.net/~schwcof/ptsd.html
PTSD Bibliography

An annotated list of books and articles about the emotional aftershocks of rape, incest, child abuse, street crime, family violence, war, Holocaust, racial violence, political terror, and other forms of psychological trauma.

http://www.mentalhealth.com/dis-rs3/p26-an06.html
PTSD: Research regarding Cause

Summaries of research studies regarding the cause of PTSD.

http://www.mentalhealth.com/dis-rs1/p24-an06.html
PTSD: Research regarding Diagnosis

Summaries of research studies regarding the diagnosis of PTSD.

http://www.mentalhealth.com/dis-rs2/p25-an06.html
PTSD: Research regarding Treatment

Summaries of research studies regarding the treatment of PTSD.

http://www.umdnj.edu/psyevnts/ptsd.html
PTSD Resources ★

Compiled by Myron Pulier. Hyperlinks references are made to the PTSD Index, the National Center for PTSD, Baldwin's Trauma Information Pages, Traumatology, Green Cross.

http://pubnet.nwu.edu/~loa773/trauma.html
Rape Trauma Syndrome
> Good explanation of the RTS (Rape Trauma Syndrome) review-
> ing the phases experienced by the survivor.

http://www.spr.org/docs/rts.html
Rape Trauma Syndrome in Male Prisoners
> Discussion by Stephen Donaldson about this devastating form
> of PTSD. While it was first discerned and described in connec-
> tion with female victims, males experience the same problem
> but have additional issues to deal with specific to their gender,
> which adds to the traumatization.

http://www.xroads.com/rahome/rahome.html
Ritual Abuse, Ritual Crime, and Healing Home Page ★
> Designed to offer support, information, and encouragement to
> survivors and to make information available to all who are
> interested in this field. Many hyperlinks.

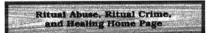

http://www.rossinst.com/
Ross Institute for Psychological Trauma ★
> The Ross Institute was formed to further the understanding of
> psychological trauma and its consequences by providing edu-
> cational services, research, and clinical treatment of trauma-
> based disorders. Valuable hyperlinks.

http://www.cs.utk.edu/~bartley/saInfoPage.html
Sexual Assault Information Page ★★
> Excellent hyperlinks to every component of sexual asault.
> Important resources for professionals and students in this
> field.

http://www.teleport.com/~snapmail/index.html
SNAP: Survivors Network of those Abused by Priests
Chicago, Illinois

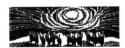

SNAP

Survivors Network of

those Abused by Priests

> A U.S.A./Canadian self-help organization of men and women
> who were sexually abused by spiritual elders. Members find
> healing and empowerment by joining with other survivors.

http://users.lanminds.com/~eds/article.html
Somatic Trauma Therapy
> An annotated trauma case history by body-psychotherapist
> Babette Rothschild indicating that there is a growing body of
> literature on PTSD showing physiological as well as psycho-
> logical elements. Case is presented illustrating this connection
> and demonstrating a sampling of techniques that address, sup-
> port, and heal this connection as a part of an integrated therapy
> for treatment of trauma.

http://psy.uq.edu.au/PTSD/trauma/trauma.html
Traumatic Stress Forum Home Page

> A forum founded by Charles Figley of Florida State University.Members study or treat those who have or are still experiencing the effects of a traumatic event. Forum's immediate concern is seeking the most powerful, painless, and efficient method for eliminating unwanted consequences of traumatic events.

http://users.lanminds.com/~eds/manual.html
Trauma Treatment Manual

> Edward Schmookler presents a manual originally written for people working with women survivors of rape in Bosnia, but able to be used more broadly as a guide for helping anyone of either gender who has survived any trauma.

http://redwood.northcoast.com/~dka/studies.htm
Treating Sexually Abused Children ★

> Presents disturbing information about effectiveness of traditional approaches. The study examined maternal mental health status and found that the mother's mental health status was the best predictor of psychological or behavioral impairment in victimized children.

http://www.lbjlib.utexas.edu/shwv/link-faq.html
Vietnam-Related Resources on WWW ★

> John Tegtmeier presents FAQ listing Vietnam-related Internet sites. Extremely comprehensive and an absolute must for anyone working in the field.

Welcome to
VOICES IN ACTION

www.voices-action.org

Victims Of Incest Can Emerge Survivors

VOICES in Action, Inc. is an international organization to provide assistance to victims of incest and child sexual abuse in becoming survivors and to generate public awareness of the prevalence of incest.

http://www.voices-action.org/
Voices in Action: Victims of Incest Can Emerge Survivors ★
Chicago, Illinois

> An international organization providing assistance to victims of incest and child sexual abuse in becoming survivors and generating public awareness of the prevalence of incest. Good hyperlinks.

http://idealist.com/wounded_healer/
Wounded Healer Journal ★

> Sponsored by Linda Champan, the Journal is a resource for survivors of childhood trauma and abuse. Many hyperlinks and newsgroups.

The
Wounded Healer Journal

Points of Departure for Psychotherapists
and Others On the Healing Journey

BOOKSTORE - RESOURCE BANK

Allies	Article Archives
"FMS" Info from Ken Pope, Ph.D. 1996 ~ 1997	Friends of TWHJ
In Crisis?	Jukebox

F. *Anxiety Disorders*

http://www.1010.com/anxiety
Anxiety and Hypoglycemia Study Group
New York, New York
> Founded in 1994 to help people learn about the most common causes of biochemical imbalance: reactive hypoglycemia, food allergy, nutritional deficiencies, toxins, and infections.

http://www.thebody.com/nimh/anxiety.html
Anxiety Disorders: Decade of the Brain ★
> Lengthy article offering brief explanation of generalized anxiety disorder, panic disorder, specific phobias, social phobias, obsessive-compulsive disorder, and posttraumatic stress disorder.

http://www.nimh.nih.gov/publicat/anxiety.htm
Anxiety Disorders: NIHM ★
> Excellent reviews of generalized anxiety disorder, panic disorder, phobias, OCD, PTSD, and how to get help.

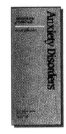

ANXIETY DISORDERS

Generalized Anxiety Disorder

Panic Disorder

Phobias

Obsessive-Compulsive Disorder

Post-Traumatic Stress Disorder

How to Get Help for Anxiety Disorder

For More Information

http://www.bu.edu/ANXIETY
Center for Anxiety and Related Disorders
Boston, Massachussetts
> Center is nationally known for assessment and treatment of anxiety disorders. Specializes in treatment and scientific investigation of phobias, other anxiety-based problems, and depression. Partially funded by grants from NIMH and National Institute of Drug Abuse.

http://www.stressrelease.com
Center for Anxiety and Stress Treatment
> Resources (books, audiotapes, etc.) to help people experiencing anxiety, stress, panic, and phobias manage and regain control of their lives.

 Center for Anxiety & Stress Treatment

Anxiety? Stress? Panic? Phobias? Worry?

Our resources can help you manage and regain control of your life.

http://www.mentalhealth.com/dis1/p21-an07.html
Generalized Anxiety Disorder: American Description
> Diagnostic criteria and associated features for generalized anxiety disorder.

http://www.mentalhealth.com/dx/dx-an07.html
Generalized Anxiety Disorder: Diagnosis
> Brief review of criteria for diagnosis. Questionnaire aids in psychiatric diagnosis.

http://www.mentalhealth.com/rx/p23-an07.html
Generalized Anxiety Disorder: Treatment
> Discusses medical and psychosocial treatments.

National Anxiety Foundation

http://www.lexington-on-line.com/naf.html
National Anxiety Foundation ★
Lexington, Kentucky
> Valuable links to information on panic disorder and OCD. Also offers references to a Directory of Anxiety Health Care Professionals.

http://www.geocities.com/HotSprings/1497
Umbra's Haven for Anxiety/Panic Disorders Survivors
> A homepage dedicated to reducing the silent suffering of people dealing with Panic and Anxiety Disorders. Silver Umbra experienced these personally and offers Umbra's story and poetry, public forums including meet the docs and ask the docs, and a pen pal panic list.

G. *Other Anxiety Resources*

http://www.stresspress.com/car/
Car-Auto-Traffic Accident Family Web Site ★
The Stress Press
> An online stress test, how-to sections, and stories from families who have recovered from crashes.

http://home.earthlink.net/~omega8/
Driving Yourself Crazy
> The "Driving Therapist" presents tapes designed to help people handle fears, stresses, or phobias associated with driving a vehicle.

http://www.mother.com/JestHome/ANTI-STRESS.HTML
Humor: An Antidote for Stress
> Good article describing research showing that humor can stimulate the immune system, enhance perceptual flexibility, and renew spiritual energy.

http://www.stressed.com/
Humor Potential, Inc.
> A site filled with resources, products, and seminars for stress reduction. References to a speakers' bureau.

The Humor Potential

Welcome to the Web Site of The Humor Potential!

A Loretta LaRoche Co.

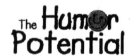

Our site is filled with resources, products and seminars for stress reduction.

Enjoy your visit to our site and let us help you discover "How to Prevent Hardening of the Attitude!"   Humor Yourself!

http://ourworld.compuserve.com/homepages/lifeline/

Lifeline

A newsletter for people and their families who suffer from the panic brought about by fears, anxieties, and phobias. Lifeline is a nonprofit quarterly publication written and published by victims of irrational panic and their families and friends. Free subscription.

http://stresscenter.com/

The Midwest Center for Stress and Anxiety

Oak Harbor, Ohio

Offers "Attacking Anxiety," a popular home-study course.

http://www.option.org/stress.html

The Option Institute

Sheffield, Massachsetts

A residential center. Offers books and tapes.

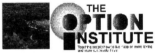

[The Option Institute | Program Listing Free Offer]

http://www.mediconsult.com/stress/drugs/index.html

Stress Drug Information

Reviews brand names, generic names, and general categories of drugs used to reduce stress. Also offers a keyword search.

http://www.pacificcoast.net/~kstrong/

Support for Support People

Information and support for family and friends to those experiencing anxiety diseases. Many links to FAQ, anxiety in the workplace, anxiety and the student, etc.

**SUPPORT PEOPLE NEED
UNDERSTANDING FRIENDS TOO .**

SUPPORT FOR SUPPORT PEOPLE

information and support for family and friends of those with anxiety diseases

H. *Mailing Lists*

Anxiety
listserv@maelstrom.stjohns.edu
SUBSCRIBE ANS-DIS

Anxiety Support
listserv@home.ease.lsoft.com
sub ANXIETY Your Name

Bodies-Under-Siege (BUS): Support for those who self injure
majordomo@majordomo.pobox.com
SUBSCRIBE BUS

Obsessive Compulsive Disorder List
listserv@vm.marist.edu
SUBSCRIBE OCD-L

Panic Disorders
Panic-Request@gnu.ai.mit.edu
COMMAND

Traumatic Stress
mailbase@mailbase.ac.uk
COMMAND

Somatoform Disorders

The common feature of Somatoform Disorders is the presence of physical symptoms suggesting a general medical condition not fully explained by a general medical condition, the direct results of a substance, or another mental disorder. These symptoms cause significant distress and impairment in everyday functioning.

The *DSM-IV* categorizes these into:

A. Somatization Disorder, beginning before age 30 and characterized by combinations of pain, gastrointestinal, sexual, and psychoneurological symptoms

B. Conversion Disorder, involving unexplained symptoms affecting voluntary motor or sensory function suggesting a neurological or medical condition.

C. Pain Disorder, in which pain is the major focus of clinical attention. Psychological factors may play a significant role.

D. Hypochondriasis, which is the preoccupation with the fear of having a serious disease based on a misinterpretation of bodily functions or symptoms

E. Body Dysmorphic Disorder, which is a preoccupation with an imagined or exaggerated defect in physical appearance.

A. *Somatization Disorder (including PTSD)*

http://www.gulfweb.org/doc_show.cfm?ID=416
Misdiagnosis of Somatization Disorder
Discusses the misdiagnosis of somatization disorder in Gulf War veterans and others with overlapping disorders of chronic fatigue, fibromyalgia, and multiple chemical sensitivity.

B. *Conversion Disorder*

http://www.mc.vanderbilt.edu/peds/pidl/adolesc/convreac.html
Conversion and Somatization Disorders
Discusses incidence and prevalence, theories, and medical illnesses predisposing people to this disorder, typical conversion symptoms, etc.

C. *Pain Disorder (including Migraine Headaches)*

http://www.achenet.org/
American Council for Headache Education ★
Woodbury, New Jersey

American Council for Headache Education

A Non-Profit Physician-Patient Partnership to Advance Headache Prevention and Treatment

> A nonprofit patient/physician partnership providing support for sufferers of chronic headache as well as offering education about this illness. ACHE produces a newsletter, brochures, video and other educational materials. Contains hyperlinks to prevention and treatment resources, physician referrals, etc.

http://weber.u.washington.edu/~crc/
Chapman's Home Page ★

> Good resource for people working in the field of pain research as well as clinicians concerned with pain control. Contains useful hyperlinks and WWW resources for pain researchers and clinicians.

http://www.migrainehelp.com/
Migraine Resource Center ★

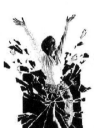

GlaxoWellcome

Migraine Resource Center

▶ WELCOME TO THE
GLAXO WELLCOME
MIGRAINE RESOURCE
CENTER.

WELCOME
WHAT IS IT?
DIAGNOSIS
SUPPORT
IMITREX
COPING
LITERATURE

> The Glaxo Wellcome Migraine Resource Center discusses triggers, symptoms, and treatment programs for migraine sufferers. Offers a free detailed diagnostic screening and a resource of support materials.

D. *Hypochrondriasis*

http://www.iop.bpmf.ac.uk/home/depts/prt/leaflets/17hyp.htm
Hypochrondriasis

> Discusses frequency, etiology, cost, management, research and conclusions. From the U.K.

E. *Body Dysmorphic Disorder*

http://www.grovelands.co.uk/bddinfo.html
Body Dysmorphic Disorder: Questions and Answers

Body Image

search
talk to others
write to us
Body & Soul

**Do You Have a
Body Image Problem?**

> Good article explaining BDD, when a physical concern becomes BDD, common areas of the body involved, the frequency of BDD, etc.

http://homearts.com/depts/health/12bodqz1.htm
Body Dysmorphic Disorder Quiz

> A brief screening test that can help people find out whether their feelings about appearance are normal concerns.

http://www.butler.org/bdd.html
Butler Body Image Program
Providence, Rhode Island

> Katherine Phillips discusses body dysmorphic disorder and offers a free evaluation for adults, adolescents, and children. Also offers free treatment for adults.

F. *Other (including Chronic Fatigue Syndrome)*

http://www.cfids.org/
CFIDS Association of America ★
Charlotte, North Carolina
> Rationale of the Association; information about news and advocacy; the CFIDS Chronicle; pediatric CFIDS; educational materials and online resources.

http://www.fnmedcenter.com/ccis
Cheney Clinic Information: Chronic Fatigue ★
Charlotte, North Carolina
> This oldest and largest clinic in the U.S. specializing in chronic fatigue syndrome. Offers an online test, FAQ, references and resources. Excellent for professionals working in the field.

http://www.lifelines.com:80/cfstxt.html
Chronic Fatigue Syndrome: Comprehensive Approach to Definition and Study ★
> Extensive article citing information from international centers that have developed a conceptual framework and set of research guidelines for use in the study of CFS. The full text of the paper from the United States Center for Disease Control.

http://www.cais.com/cfs-news/
Chronic Fatigue Syndrome: FAQ ★
> Very comprehensive resource discussing every aspect of chronic fatigue syndrome. Invaluable for professionals and students in the field.

http://www2.lainet.com/~simonton/
Simonton Cancer Center: Aspects of Mind-Body Medicine
Pacific Palisades, California
> Often described as a trailblazer and pioneer in psychoneuroimmunology, Dr. Simonton is Founder and Medical Director of the Simonton Cancer Center in California. Books and tapes are available as well as patient programs and patient resources.

Stanford University School of Medicine
Department of Psychiatry and Behavioral Sciences
Psychosocial Treatment Laboratory

http://www-med.stanford.edu/school/Psychiatry/PSTreatLab/ms.html
Stanford University Psychosocial Treatment Lab
> From the Stanford Department of Psychiatry and Behavioral Science. The mission statement is explained, as well as the metastatic study, research with cancer and HIV, trauma, hypnosis, and much more.

G. *Mailing List*

Chronic Pain
listserv@maelstrom.stjohns.edu
SUBSCRIBE PAIN-L Your Name

Factitious Disorders

Factitious Disorders are characterized by physical or psychological symptoms intentionally produced or feigned in order to assume the sick role. The essential feature is the intentional production of symptoms of sickness. The motivation is assumption of the sick role.

Factitious Disorders *per se* are not represented on the Internet. Factitious Disorders by Proxy are listed in the *DSM-IV* as a disorder for further study. Munchausen Syndrome best fits this category and is represented on the Internet.

A. *Munchausen Syndrome*

http://www.ncjrs.org/txtfiles/chnegmun.txt
Child Neglect and Munchausen Syndrome by Proxy
> Lengthy article from the U.S. Department of Justice discussing child neglect and Munchausen syndrome.

http://www.merck.com/!!uMww6264luMwyB2bx6/pubs/
mmanual/html/nimldge.htm
Merck Manual: Munchausen Syndrome
> Discusses Munchausen syndrome and dynamics involved. Excellent article from a psychiatric viewpoint. Also alludes to Munchausen by proxy.

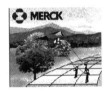

http://www.merck.com/!!uMww6264luMwyB2bx6/pubs/
mmanual/html/nimldge.htm
Merck Manual: Munchausen Syndrome, Treatment
> Brief comments on treatment and potential success with Munchausen syndrome.

http://www.msbp.com/
Mothers Against Munchausen Syndrome by Proxy Allegations
> MAMA's mission is to stop the assault on innocent mothers and fathers from false accusations and to reveal the ulterior motives of the accusers.

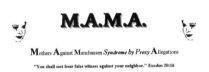

M.A.M.A.

Mothers Against Munchausen *Syndrome by Proxy* Allegations

"You shall not bear false witness against your neighbor." Exodus 20:16

http://ourworld.compuserve.com/homepages/Marc_Feldman_2/
Munchausen Syndrome and Factitious Disorder Page ★
> Psychiatrist Dr. Marc Feldman discusses Munchausen syndrome and other factitious disorders. Excellent resource. Contains hyperlinks.

http://www.kfshrc.edu.sa/annals/154/94280/94280.html
Munchausen Syndrome Presenting as Immunodeficiency
> A case report and review of literature.

SECTION X.
Dissociative Disorders (including False Memory Syndrome)

Describing the essential feature of Dissociative Disorders, the *DSM-IV* indicates a disruption in the usually integrated functions of consciousness, memory, identity, or perception of the environment. The disorders are divided into:

A. Dissociative Amnesia, characterized by inability to recall important personal information too extensive to be explained by ordinary forgetfulness.
B. Dissociative Fugue, characterized by sudden and unexplainable travel away from familiar places and accompanied by inability to recall one's past.
C. Dissociative Identity Disorder (formerly Multiple Personality Disorder), characterized by the presence of two or more distinct identities or personality states.
D. Depersonalization Disorder, characterized by a persistent feeling of being detached from one's mental processes or body.

While not a *DSM-IV* disorder, False Memory Syndrome is currently a topic receiving a great deal of attention in the mental health community. Resources for False Memory Syndrome are listed in this section.

A. *Dissociative Amnesia*

http://www.cmhc.com/disorders/sx46.htm
Dissociative Amnesia: Symptoms
  Brief description of symptoms of dissociative amnesia.

B. *Dissociative Fugue*

http://www.cmhc.com/disorders/sx87.htm
Dissociative Fugue: Symptoms
  Brief description of symptoms of dissociative fugue.

C. *Dissociative Identity Disorder*

http://wchat.on.ca/web/asarc/mpd.html
Child Abuse and Multiple Personality Disorder
> By Philip Coons. Reviews the syndrome of multiple personality associated with physical and or sexual abuse in childhood. Describes the history, clinical features, and treatment of multiple personality, particularly in children, in addition to exploring the professional reluctance to make the diagnosis.

http://www.sidran.org/didbr.html
Dissociative Identity Disorder (Multiple Personality Disorder)
> Brochure by Sidran Foundation explaining this disorder.

http://www.cmhc.com/disorders/sx18.htm
Dissociative Identity Disorder: Symptoms
> Brief explanation of symptoms of dissociative identity disorder.

http://www.cmhc.com/disorders/sx18t.htm
Dissociative Identity Disorder: Treatment
> Psychotherapy, medications and self-help resources for MPD.

http://www.dhearts.org/
Divided Hearts: DID/MPD Info and Support Web ★
> Offers interactive forums, library resources, stress and suicide pages, and suggestions on how to get involved. Many hyperlinks.

http://www.issd.org/isdguide.htm
Guidelines for Treating Dissociative Identity Disorder
> From the International Society for the Study of Dissociation, the guidelines present a broad outline of what seems to be effective in the treatment of DID.

http://qlink.queensu.ca/~3jgb2/mpd.html
Multiple Personality and Dissociative Disorders
> Good overview of facts, symptoms, terms, etc., regarding MPD

http://www.vuw.ac.nz/~anita/dissociation.html
Multiple Personality Disorder and Dissociation Resources ★
> Resource list on dissociation and MPD. Contains book listings and hyperlinks.

http://slt.pobox.com/revenge/mpd.html
Multiple Personality Disorder Dispute
> Good analysis of the ongoing debate between MPD and false memory syndrome adherents.

Sidran Home | News | About | Resources | Bookshelf | E-Mail

TRAUMA RESOURCE AREA

Dissociative Identity Disorder (Multiple Personality Disorder)

DividedHearts
DID/MPD Info & Support Web

MULTIPLE PERSONALITY RESOURCES

http://www.asarian.org/~astraea/household/
Unorthodox Multiple Personality Resources ★★
> References to social and political issues, online support and chat groups, newsgroups, mailing lists, and SANCTUARY.

D. *Depersonalization Disorder*

http://www.xs4all.nl/~mauricex/depers/
Depersonalization Disorder Page
> Maurice Hendrix from Holland, who suffers from a depersonalization disorder, exchanges information about how depersonalization disorder controls one's life, coping strategies, useful medications, and other useful information.

E. *Other (including False Memory Syndrome)*

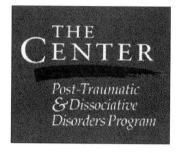

http://www.voiceofwomen.com/VOW2_11950/center.html
Center for Post-Traumatic and Dissociative Disorders
Washington, D.C.
> Offering short-term directed treatment for adults with dissociative disorders resulting from childhood tauma. Training in self-management skills using cognitive-behavioral strategies.

http://adhostnt.adhost.com/cgi-win/athealth32.exe?12
Dissociative Disorders
> Describes the main characteristics for each dissociative disorder.

The False Memory Syndrome Foundation

While our awareness of childhood sexual abuse has increased enormously in the last decade and the horrors of its consequences should never be minimized, there is another side to this situation, namely that of the consequences of false allegations where whole families are split apart and terrible pain inflicted on everyone concerned. This side of the story needs to be told, for a therapist may, with the best intentions in the world, contribute to enormous family suffering.
-- Harold Lief, M.D.

http://advicom.net/~fitz/fmsf/
False Memory Syndrome Foundation ★
> Describes FMS, the Foundation, mailing lists, and articles, as well as events.

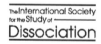

TheInternational Society
for the Study of ——————
Dissociation **Home Page**

The ISSD brings together professionals dedicated to the search for answers to improve the quality of life for all patients with dissociative disorders.

http://www.issd.org/
International Society for the Study of Dissociation
Glenview, Illinois
> An international non-profit society that promotes research and training, professional and public education, and international communication and cooperation among clinicians working in the field of dissociation.

http://www.geocities.com/HotSprings/4514
Minnesota Awareness of Ritual Abuse Network ★
> Provides education about ritual abuse and its harmful impact on society. Seeks to dispel societal myths about victims and survivors of ritual abuse.

http://www.jimhopper.com/memory
Recovered Memories of Sexual Abuse: Research and Resources ★
> Extensive resource discussing empirical evidence, psychological constructs, research findings and scientific progress.

http://members.aol.com/SRAHaven/
Safe Haven for Satanic Ritual Abuse and Survivors ★
> Unusual resource attempting to create a safe haven for survivors of satanic ritual abuse, mind control victims, brain implant victims, military or torture programming victims, and those coping with a dissociative condition.

Welcome to a caring forum for Satanic Ritual Abuse/Ritual Abuse Survivors, Mind Control Survivors, and/or those facing a Dissociative Condition such as MPD/DID.

http://www.asarian.org/
Survivors of Sexual Abuse ★
> A service to survivors of sexual abuse. Many hyperlinks.

http://ourworld.compuserve.com/homepages/Synergy_
Institute_npo
Synergy: Institute for Dissociative Disorders ★
> California-based non-profit institute whose mission is to provide information, research, and education to the professional community and general public.

F. *Mailing Lists*

Dissociative Disorders Discussion
listserv@maelstrom.stjohns.edu
SUBSCRIBE DISSOCIATIVE-DISORDERS

DID/MPD/Sexual Abuse Support Group
listserv@maelstrom.stjohns.edu
SUBSCRIBE SADM

Sexual and Gender Identity Disorders (also includes Gay, Lesbian, Bisexual and Transgendered Issues Not Considered a Disorder)

Sexual Disorders fall into three categories:

A. Sexual Dysfunctions, characterized by disturbances in the processes of the sexual response cycle or by pain associated with sexual intercourse.

B. Paraphilias, characterized by recurrent, intense sexual urges, fantasies, or behaviors that involve unusual objects, activities, or situations that cause significant distress or impairment in normal functioning.

C. Gender Identity Disorders, characterized by strong and persistent cross-gender identification accompanied by persistent discomfort with one's assigned sex.

Homosexuality, bisexuality, and transsexualism are not considered psychological or psychiatric disorders. This has been the American Psychiatric Association and American Psychological Association position for decades. However, gays, lesbians, bisexuals and transgendered individuals are very active on the Internet, providing valuable sites for clinicians as well as for members of their community. Inclusion of these sites is intended to help people cope with the stigma and stress that often accompany being different. In order to offer this extremely valuable information to clinicians and ultimately to their clients, we have placed these sites in a separate section entitled "E. Sexual Orientation Issues and Conditions Not Considered Disorders."

A. *Sexual Dysfunctions*

i. *SEXUAL DESIRE DISORDERS (HYPOACTIVE; SEXUAL AVERSION)*

Sexual Disorders

http://adhostnt.adhost.com/cgi-win/athealth32.exe?31
Sexual Disorders
Discusses sexual dysfunctions, giving examples of many types of dysfunctions.

ii. SEXUAL AROUSAL DISORDERS (FEMALE AROUSAL DISORDERS; MALE ERECTILE DISORDERS)

http://www.pslgroup.com/dg950830.htm
Caverject to Treat Impotence
>   Caverject is the first prescription medication cleared for marketing as a treatment for erectile dysfunction. Discusses Caverject, how administered and the impact on impotence.

http://www.for-men.com/
Diagnostic Center for Men
>   A nationwide network of specialty medical clinics that exclusively evaluate and treat men with sexual dysfunctions. 25 diagnostic centers are located in the U.S.

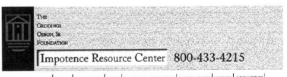

http://h-devil-www.mc.duke.edu/h-devil/men/dysfunct.htm
Erectile Dysfunction
>   Lists physical, psychological, and interpersonal causes of erectile dysfunction.

http://text.nlm.nih.gov/nih/cdc/www/91txt.html
Impotence ★
>   Lengthy text of the National Institutes of Health Consensus Development Conference on Impotence held in December 1992. Offers a summary of findings.

http://www.medicdrug.com/impotence/
impotence.html
Impotence Information Center
>   Provides comprehensive information on impotence, and information on all currently acceptable FDA approved treatments.

http://www.impotence.org/
Impotence Resource Center
>   A non-profit organization dedicated to improving the quality of life by promoting a better understanding of sensitive medical disorders.

http://www.cmhc.com/disorders/sx59.htm
Male Erectile Disorder: Symptoms
>   Brief description of symptoms of male erectile disorder.

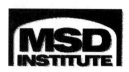

This is a message of hope. Impotence is curable. No man need suffer the shame, the torment and the agony of impotence because with the present state of the art, nearly every man can be cured. Twenty million American men, both young and old, are afflicted with this problem. At the MSD Institute our youngest patient is 17 and our oldest is 92. Tragically, fewer than 5% seek help. Help is available and affordable. Impotence is curable!

http://www.msdinst.com
MSD Institute
Chicago, Illinois
> Devoted to the diagnosis and treatment of impotence. Maintains a 24-hour hot line at (800) 788-CURE

http://bestsex.com/Vol5.html
Overcoming Sexual Problems
> A videotape by a psychiatrist who is a sex therapist. Explores the causes of sexual problems. The tape answers questions and demonstrates methods to help correct sexual dysfunctions.

http://eee.oac.uci.edu/96s/class/p121da/dysfunc.html
Sexual Dysfunction ★
> Discusses female sexual dysfunction, male sexual dysfunction, and their causes. Offers case examples.

http://www.zplace.com/numedtec/
Successfully Treating Impotence
> Attempts to dispel the myths, uncover interesting facts, and answer FAQ about impotence. Focuses on successful treatment of impotence.

iii. ORGASMIC DISORDERS (FEMALE, MALE; PREMATURE EJACULATION)

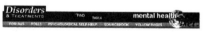

Female and Male Orgasmic Disorders
SYMPTOMS

http:www.cmch.com/disorders/sx58.htm
Female and Male Orgasmic Disorders
> Lists symptoms of female and male orgasmic disorder.

http://h-devil-www.mc.duke.edu/h-devil/men/ejac.htm
Premature Ejaculation
> Brief article describing premature ejaculation and tips for what a person can do about this condition.

http://www.cmhc.com/disorders/sx64.htm
Premature Ejaculation: Symptoms
> Brief description of symptoms of premature ejaculation. Links to treatment and online resources.

http://www.cmhc.com/disorders/sx64t.htm
Premature Ejaculation: Treatment
> Discusses psychotherapy, medications and self-help programs.

http://www.personal.u-net.com/~shmid/premauk.htm
Premature Ejaculation Annihilated
> Discusses the nature of the problem, frequency in males, physiological vs. psychological basis, etc.

iv. SEXUAL PAIN DISORDERS (DYSPAREUNIA, VAGINISMUS)

http://www.cmhc.com/disorders/sx49.htm
Dyspareunia: Symptoms
Describes symptoms of dyspareunia.
http://incontinet.com/articles/art_sex/vaginis.htm
Treating Vaginismus with Perry brand sensors
Insertable EMG pelvic muscle sensors for patients having a penetration problem.

http://www.cmhc.com/disorders/sx97.htm
Vaginismus
Describes symptoms of vaginismus.

B. *Paraphilias*

i. Exhibitionism, a disorder where one obtains sexual arousal by exposing genitals to unsuspecting strangers.
ii. Fetishism, a disorder where one obtains sexual arousal by thinking about an inanimate object or part of the body.
iii. Pedophilia, a disorder where one obtains sexual arousal and gratification through sexual activity or fantasizing about having sexual activity with children who have not reached puberty.
iv. Sexual Masochism, a disorder where one obtains sexual arousal and gratification by having pain and/or humiliation inflicted upon oneself.
v. Sexual Sadism, a disorder where one obtains sexual arousal and gratification primarily or exclusively by inflicting pain on another person.
vi. Transvestic Fetishism, a disorder where one obtains sexual arousal by thinking about an inanimate object or a particular part of the body.
vii. Voyeurism, a disorder where one obtains sexual arousal by observing nude individuals without their knowledge or consent (a Peeping Tom).

http://adhostnt.adhost.com/cgi-win/athealth32.exe?24
Paraphilias
Discusses the common paraphilias, including age at onset and treatment options.

http://andes.ip.ucsb.edu/~satyr/philia/index.html
Paraphilia Resource Page
Lists paraphilias alphabetically. Hyperlinks to many of these for more information. Attempts to present an educational and entertaining glimpse into humanity's psychosexual potential.

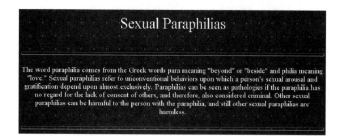

The word paraphilia comes from the Greek words para meaning "beyond" or "beside" and philia meaning "love." Sexual paraphilias refer to unconventional behaviors upon which a person's sexual arousal and gratification depend upon almost exclusively. Paraphilias can be seen as pathologies if the paraphilia has no regard for the lack of consent of others, and therefore, also considered criminal. Other sexual paraphilias can be harmful to the person with the paraphilia, and still other sexual paraphilias are harmless.

http://www.public.asu.edu/~ide4bubu/sexlinks/philia.html
Sexual Paraphilias
Describes sexual paraphilias, with links to additional symptoms. Contains a reading list for further information.

http://www.mhsource.com/edu/psytimes/p960627.html
Therapy for Sexual Impulsivity
Excellent overview of sexual impulse disorders by Martin Kafka.

C. *Gender Identity Disorders*

http://www.3dcom.com/tg/gic/what.html
Gender Identity Center
Lakewood, Colorado
Colorado-based program providing support, information, and referrals to transgendered people, their families and friends, and education to the community at large.

http://www.genderweb.org/
Gender Identity Clinic ★★
Extensive links to transgendered phenomena, diagnosis and care, transition and transformation, support services, reassignment surgery, etc.

http://adhostnt.adhost/com/cgi-win/athealth32.exe?15
Gender Identity Disorder
Discusses gender identity; characteristics and male/female ratio, age of onset, diagnosis, etc.

http://www.cmhc.com/disorders/sx40.htm
Gender Identity Disorders: Symptoms
DSM-IV criteria discussing symptoms of gender identity disorder.

D. *Other Sites of General Interest*

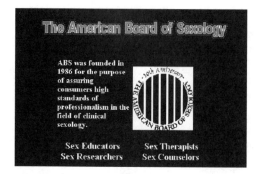

http://www.indiana.edu/~kinsey/ABS/newhome.html
American Board of Sexology
Founded in 1985 for the purpose of assuring high standards of professionalism in the field of clinical sexology. Discusses certification requirements and information regarding finding a therapist.

http://www.med.nyu.edu/Psych/screens/sdsm.html
Online Sexual Disorders Screening for Men
> Sexual questionnaire developed by NYU Department of Psychiatry.

http://www.med.nyu.edu/Psych/screens/sdsf.html
Online Sexual Disorders Screening for Women
> Sexual questionnaire developed by NYU Department of Psychiatry.

http://www.priory.com/sex.htm
Sexual Disorders
> Comprehensive article on sexual disorders. Includes an overview of the *DSM-IV* criteria, a table dealing with the physical causes of male erectile failure, a table dealing with causes of dyspareunia, estimated prevalence of sexual problems in young adults, what can be done.

http://www.usrf.org/
Urological Sciences Research Foundation
> A California not-for-profit organization to "help advance the understanding of common urologic problems."

E. *Sexual Orientation Issues and Conditions Not Considered Disorders*

http://www.ren.org/rafil/aegis.html
AEGIS Information Center ★
Decatur, Georgia
> Successor to the Erikson Educational Foundation. Provides educational resources for professionals and transgendered persons. Maintains a database of free professional services.

http://host2.mbcomms.net.au/austg/
Australasian Good Tranny Guide ★
> Discusses social and supports groups, medical services, legal services, and tranny-friendly business in Australia and New Zealand.

http://www.geocities.com/WestHollywood/1769/pride.html
Beverly's Homepage: Lesbian, Gay, Bisexual and Transvestite Resources ★
> Beverly's thoughts and resources for LGBT community. Many hyperlinks.

http://www.deafqueer.org/
Deaf Queer Resource Center
> Promotes deaf queer visibility on the web.

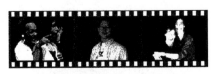

"Proudly promoting Deaf Queer visibility on the Web!"

http://www.savina.com/confluence/hormone/
FAQ: Hormone Therapy for Transsexuals ★
>Extensive information about gonadal hormones and hormones for the treatment of androgen and estrogen-sensitive conditions.Questions and answers available in English, Italian, and Swedish.

http://www.ftm-intl.org/intro.html
FTM International ★
>Peer support group for female-to-male transvestites and transsexuals. Many links.

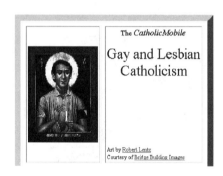

The *CatholicMobile*
Gay and Lesbian Catholicism

Art by Robert Lentz
Courtesy of Bridge Building Images

http://www.mcgill.pvt.k12.al.us/jerryd/cm/gay.htm
Gay and Lesbian Catholicism
>Links to various letters and statements regarding homosexuality and Roman Catholicism.

http://nac.adopt.org/gay/indexgay.html
Gay and Lesbian Issues
>Links to issues of lesbian and gay parenting; reference to a study indicating that lesbian couples raise psychologically healthy children; support groups for gay and lesbian parents; information specific to gay and lesbian issues in adoption.

http://www.nyu.edu/pages/sls/gaywork/gaywkpl.html
Gay Workplace Issues Homepage ★
>Discusses company policies, unions and gay employees, government and workplace issues, etc.

http://www.virtualcity.com/youthsuicide/
Gay and Bisexual Male Youth Suicidality Studies
>Hyperlinks to studies on male suicide among homosexual youth.

http://www.geocities.com/WestHollywood/1348/
Homosexuality: Common Questions and Statements Addressed ★
>Extensive resources reviewing definitions, nature/ nurture question, children and family values, civil rights, religion, and more. A must for those interested in homosexuality.

IFGE Home Page

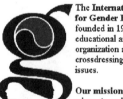

The **International Foundation for Gender Education**, founded in 1978, is an educational and charitable organization addressing crossdressing and transgender issues.

Our mission is to be the leading advocate and educational organization for

* promoting self-definition and free expression of individual gender identity;
* changing the paragidm of gender identity by recognizing the distinction between sexual orientation and gender.

To this end IFGE values:

* individual uniqueness and dignity;
* respect for human diversity;
* freedom from society's arbitrarily assigned gender definitions;
* respect, acceptance, enforcement, and protection of gender-related Human and Civil Rights.

http://www.ifge.org
International Foundation for Gender Education
Waltham, Massachusetts
>Founded in 1978, IFGT is an educational and charitable organization addressing cross-dressing and transgender issues.

http://www.isna.org/
Intersex Society of North America ★
> A peer support, education, and advocacy group founded and operated by and for intersexuals, i.e., individuals born with anatomy or physiology that differs from cultural ideals of male and female.

http://www.lesbian.org/moms
Lesbian Moms ★
> Offers a place where lesbian moms can share personal experiences, discuss issues, resources, events, and ideas.

http://www.lesbian.org/lesbian-moms/
Lesbian Mothers Support Society ★
Calgary, Alberta, Canada
> A Canadian, non-profit group that strives to provide peer support for lesbian parents and their children, as well as those lesbians considering parenthood.

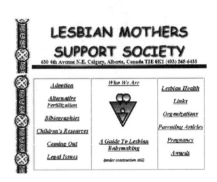

http://www.ren.org/
Renaissance Education Association
Wayne, Pennsylvania
> Founded in 1987, Renaissance provides a safe space for all transgendered people, as well as gender education for transgendered people, helping professionals, and the general public.

http://www.twentyclub.org/documents/socare.html
Standards of Care: Hormonal and Surgical Sex Reassignment ★
> Major resource detailing the standards of care for hormonal and surgical reassignment of gender dysphoric persons by the Harry Benjamin International Dysphoria Association, Inc.

http://www.savina.com/confluence/trans/
TRANS
> Founded by transsexual physicians and scientists to conduct research in areas of importance to transsexuals and other transgendered persons. Interested in examining the anatomic and physiological bases of transsexualism and gender identity. Lists members, current research, and social implications.

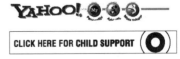

http://www.yahoo.com/Society_and_Culture/Gender/Transgendered/
Transgendered: General Resources ★★
> Many links to gender issues. Extensive resources.

http://ezinfo.ucs.indiana.edu/~mberz/ttt.html
Transvestite, Transsexual, Transgendered Homepage ★★
> Many hyperlinks to articles, songs and poetry. Referrals to newsgroups and regional resources.

WELCOME TO...

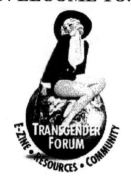

http://php.indiana.edu/~mberz/faqs.html

Transgender: Information and FAQS ★

Comprehensive resource with questions and answers dealing with every aspect of the transvestite, transsexual and transgendered community. Valuable hyperlinks.

http://www.transgender.org/

Transgender Forum

Community support groups in various cities in the U.S.

http://travesti.geophys.mcgill.ca/~tstar/

Tstar ★

Provides valuable information to the transgendered community. Includes references to sources in the U.K. and France. References to Usenet newsgroups and Internet list-services. Lists support groups, educational foundations, medical, legal, and other professional services for the transgendered community.

F. *Mailing Lists*

Bisexuality and Gender Discussion
listserv@brownvm.brown.edu
SUB BITHRY-L Your Name

Celibate Life
ebehr@internode.net
indicate a wish to join the listserv@
    maelstrom.stjohns.edu

Gender
majordomo@ifi.uio.no
SUBSCRIBE GENDER

CRUX: Sexuality Discussion
majordomo@queer.org.au
SUBSCRIBE CRUX

Society for Human Sexuality
listproc.u.washington.edu
SUBSCRIBE SHS Your Name

Transgender Issues
listserv@brownvm.brown.edu
SUBSCRIBE TRANSGEN
REVIEW TRANSGEN

Transgender Spirituality
listserv@aol.com
SUBSCRIBE TG-SPIRIT

Eating Disorders

Eating Disorders are characterized by severe disturbances in eating behavior, usually classified as Anorexia Nervosa, refusal to maintain a minimally normal body weight, or Bulimia Nervosa, characterized by repeated episodes of binge-eating followed by self-induced vomiting, use of laxatives, fasting, or excessive exercise.

A. *Anorexia Nervosa*

http://www.anred.com/
Anorexia Nervosa and Related Eating Disorders, Inc.
Eugene, Oregon
> A non-profit organization providing free and low-cost information about anorexia nervosa, bulimia nervosa, and binge-eating disorder. Materials include details about recovery and prevention.

http://www.mentalhealth.com/dis-rs3/p26-et01.html
Anorexia Nervosa: Research regarding Cause
> Summary of studies dealing with the cause of anorexia nervosa.

http://www.mentalhealth.com/rx/p23-et01.html
Anorexia Nervosa: Treatment
> Medical and psychosocial treatments.

B. *Bulimia Nervosa*

http://www.mentalhealth.com/dx/dx-et02.html
Bulimia Nervosa: Diagnosis
> Gives requirements for accurate psychiatric diagnosis and a diagnostic program.

http://www.mentalhealth.com/rx/p23-et02.html
Bulimia Nervosa: Treatment
Reviews medical and psychosocial treatments.

http://www.mentalhealth.com/dis-rsl/p24-et02.html
Research regarding Diagnosis
> Comprehensive summary of research studies dealing with the diagnosis of bulimia nervosa.

http://www.mentalhealth.com/dis-rs2/p25-et02.html
Research regarding Treatment
> Comprehensive summary of research studies dealing with treatment of bulimia nervosa.

C. *General Information and Resources for Eating Disorders*

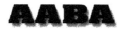

The American Anorexia/Bulimia Association, Inc.

More than five million Americans suffer from eating disorders.

Five percent of adolescent and adult women and one percent of men have anorexia nervosa, bulimia nervosa or binge-eating disorder.

Fifteen percent of young women have substantially disordered eating attitudes and behaviors.

As estimated 1,000 women die each year of anorexia nervosa.

http://members.aol.com/amanbu/index.html
American Anorexia/Bulimia Association ★
New York, New York

Association was founded to increase public consciousness of eating disorders: prevalence, warning signs and symptoms, and prevention. Provides information to sufferers, their families and friends about effective treatments.

http://www.eatright.org/anorexiainter.html
American Dietetic Association ★
Chicago, Illinois

States the position of the ADA re Nutrition Intervention in the treatment of anorexia nervosa, bulimia nervosa, and binge-eating.

http://www.stud.ntnu.no/studorg/ikstrh/ed/
Cath's Links to Eating Disorders Resources ★

A collection of links to various information on Eating Disorders on the Internet. References information in Canada, the U.K., Scandinavia, and other European sites. Also refers to some campus social/health services, various therapists and centers.

http://www.social/com/health/nhic/data/hr2100/hr2111.html
Center for the Study of Anorexia and Bulimia ★
New York, New York

Established in 1979 the Center has four objectives: effective treatment, specialized training, significant research, and increased community understanding. The Center sees anorexia and bulimia as primarily psychological disorders. Center also produces pamphlets and a teacher's health curriculum guide for grades 7 to 12 on anorexia nervosa and bulimia.

http://www.addictions.net/eating.htm
Eating Disorders ★

Links to signs and symptoms; information on pre-adolescents; treatment; guides to daily food choice; etc.

Eating Disorders

● Signs and Symptoms of an Eating Disorder	● Do's and Don'ts - For Family and Friends
● Pre-Adolescents - Regarding Body Image	● Treatment for Eating Disorders - Article
● Hidden Behind the Eating Disorder	● Contemplations for Growth
● Reading and Reference Material	● Interesting Eating Disorder Information
1. Weight Control and Exercise 2. Eating Disorders	1. History about Eating Disorders 2. Men and Eating Disorders
● Helpful Homework	● Anorexia/Bulimia Progression Chart (327K GIF)
1. Assessing Signs and Symptoms 2. Testing your Thoughts 3. Thought Distortions 4. Mis-Communications Styles	● Guide to Daily Food Choices
	1. Food Pyramid Chart (313K GIF) 2. Servings Chart (313K GIF)

http://members.aol.com/edapinc/home.html
Eating Disorders Awareness and Prevention ★
Seattle, Washington

> A national non-profit organization dedicated to increasing the awareness and prevention of eating disorders. Provides educational resources for schools, health professionals, community organizations, and interested individuals. Contains hyperlinks to many resources.

http://www.uq.edu.au/~zzedainc/n3index.html
Eating Disorders Association Resource Centre ★
Brisbane, Australia

> A source for information on eating disorders and stories from real people about real experiences.

http://www.edrecovery.com/
Eating Disorder Recovery Online
Tucson, Arizona

> Online service providing information and programs to help those recovering from a eating disorder regain self-esteem and empowerment. Developed to meet the needs of people who are unable to access or afford conventional therapy.

http://members.aol.com/mainat/pages/eat.html
Eating Right and Staying Healthy

> An online magazine dedicated to health, fitness, foods and nutrition. Formerly called Foods and Nutrition Online. Good resource!

http://194.80.201.68:80/eat_d/eced/
European Council on Eating Disorders

> Contains many hyperlinks to various newsletters. Page is hosted in the belief that psychotherapy and psychological handling remain the mainstay in the treatment of eating disorders.

http://www.per.ualberta.ca/wsi/wsitask.htm
Female Athlete Triad Task Force
Wembley, WA, Australia

> From an International Forum on the Female Athlete. Discusses eating disorders, amenorrhea, and osteoporosis. Excellent information for all female athletes and their coaches.

http://www.iop.bpmf.ac.uk./home/depts/psychiat/edu/eat.htm
Lucy Serpell's Eating/Eating Disorders Resources ★

> Many hyperlinks to all eating disorder resources. Invaluable for professionals in this field!

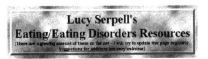

http://www.gmu.edu/gmu/personal/eating.html
Myths and Campus Resources
Fairfax, Virginia

Prepared by the Counseling Center at George Mason University, offers great commonsense information for college students. Presents myths about eating disorders and how these may prevent individuals from getting treatment.

http://www.medhelp.org/amshc/amshc40.htm
National Association of Anorexia Nervosa and Associated Disorders
Highland Park, Illinois

Provides information on self-help groups, therapy, and referrals to professionals.

NAAFA *Online*

National Association to Advance Fat Acceptance

http://naafa.org
National Association to Advance Fat Acceptance
Sacramento, California

A non-profit human rights organization dedicated to improving the quality of life for fat people. Since 1969 NAAFA has been working to eliminate discrimination based on body size and provide fat people with the tools for self-empowerment through public education, advocacy, and member support.

http://www.kidsource.com/nedo/index.html
National Eating Disorders Organization
Tulsa, Oklahoma

Founded in 1977, NEDO offers support, referral, and education for people suffering from anorexia, bulimia, and related eating disorders, their families, and friends.

http://www.weight.com/
Obesity and Weight Control ★

Michael Myers presents objective medical information on obesity/weight control, eating disorders, and other related medical conditions. References to medications and their use and effectiveness. Good hyperlinks.

http://www.iop.bpmf.ac.uk/home/depts/psychiat/edu/osteo.htm
Osteoporosis and Eating Disorders

Discusses osteoporosis and the relationship to eating disorders. Explains what osteoporosis is, how to diagnose, prevent, and treat.

http://www.angelfire.com/nm/oaregion10/index.html
Overeaters, Undereaters, Bulimics and Anorexics in Australia, New Zealand, Asia and Ocean

A fellowship of individuals from all walks of life who meet in order to help solve a range of eating disorders.

http://www.hiwaay.net/recovery/
Overeaters Recovery Group Home Page ★

An organization of individuals who, through shared experience, strength, and hope, are recovering from compulsive eating. While many subscribe to the 12-Step program, this is not a requirement. Contains hyperlinks to various services.

http://www.renfrew.org/
Renfrew Center

A woman's mental health center with many locations and a nationwide referral network. Specializes in treatment of eating disorder, trauma, anxiety, depression, substance abuse, and other women's issues.

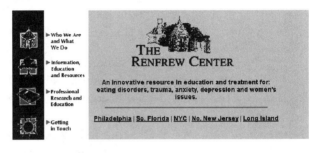

http://pharminfo.com/pubs/msb/seroton.html
Serotonin and Eating Disorders

From *Medical Sciences Bulletin*. Discusses serotonin and eating disorders.

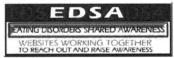

http://www.eating-disorder.com
Something Fishy Website on Eating Disorders ★

Excellent page with hyperlinks dealing with all issues of eating disorders. Winner of many mental health awards.

D. *Mailing Lists*

Eating Disorders Discussion
listserv@maelstrom.stjohns.edu
SUBSCRIBE EATING-DISORDERS

Overeaters Recovery Group
listserv@maelstrom.stjohns.edu
SUBSCRIBE OASIS

Primary sleep disorders are divided into dyssomnias (abnormalities in the amount, quality, or timing of sleep) and parasomnias (abnormal behavior or physiological events occurring in association with sleep, sleep stages, or sleep-wake transition).

A. Dyssomnias
    i. Insomnia. Difficulty initiating or maintaining sleep, or non-restorative sleep, lasting for at least 1 month.
    ii. Hypersomnia. Excessive sleepiness for at least 1 month, as evidenced by prolonged sleep episodes or daytime sleep episodes occurring almost daily.
    iii. Narcolepsy. Irresistible attacks of refreshing sleep that occur daily over a 3-month period.
    iv. Breathing-related Sleep Disorder. Sleep disruption leading to excessive sleepiness or insomnia.
    v. Circadian Rhythm Sleep Disorder. Persistent or recurrent pattern of sleep disruption leading to excessive sleepiness or insomnia that is due to a mismatch between the sleep-wake schedule required by someone's environment and their circadian sleep-wake pattern.
    vi. Others
    a. environmental factors
    b. sleep deprivation
    c. restless leg syndrome
    d. nocturnal myoclonous (brief limb jerks)
B. Parasomnias
    i. Nightmare disorder. A repeated occurrence of frightening dreams that lead to awakenings from sleep.
    ii. Sleep Terror disorder. Abrupt awakenings from sleep usually beginning with a panicky scream or cry.
    iii. Sleepwalking disorder. Repeated episodes of complex motor behavior initiated during sleep, including rising from bed and walking about.
    iv. Others . . .
    a. motor activity
    b. sleep paralysis

A. *Dyssomnias*

i. *INSOMNIAS*

http://www.well.com/user/mick/insomnia/
Insomnia ★
> Collection of a variety of methods for falling asleep. Designed to deal with tension, stress and anxiety. Good exercises for those who think they have tried everything but nothing works.

http://www.cmhc.com/disorders/sx86.htm
Insomnia: Symptoms
> Listing of symptoms for insomnia..

http://www.sleepnet.com/
SleepNet ★★
> Attempts to link all sleep information on the net. Covers insomnias, narcolepsy, sleep apnea, restless leg syndrome, etc. Sleep links and research links are rated and reviewed. First choice for searching.

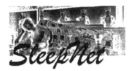

About 50 million Americans suffer from sleep disorders such as narcolepsy, sleep apnea, restless legs syndrome, and the insomnias. Most are unaware.

http://www.autonomy.com/sleep.htm
Sleep Research and Sleep Disorder Web Central ★
> Offers websites and resources on sleep, dreams, sleep disorders, and related research. Produced by Autonomy Publishing Corporation, which produces software and publishes books.

http://www-leland.stanford.edu/~dement/
Sleep Well ★★
> A reservoir of information on sleep and sleep disorders. Contains many hyperlinks to information on new developments, listings of other sleep sites, health and medical links, snoring, dreams. Offers the Epworth Sleepiness Sleep test online and contains listings of accredited sleep disorder centers in the U.S. An absolute must for researchers and clinicians.

THE SLEEP WELL

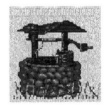

ii. *HYPERSOMNIA*

http://www.cmhc.com/disorders/sx85.htm
Hypersomnia: Symptoms
> Listing of symptoms for hypersomnia.

iii. *NARCOLEPSY*

http://www.uic.edu/depts/cnr/cindex.htm
Center for Narcolepsy Research
University of Illinois at Chicago
> In 1986, with a combination of private funding and overhead support from UI, Chicago, CNR was established to study the biobehavioral aspects of sleeping.

Center for Narcolepsy Research

University of Illinois at Chicago

http://www.cmhc.com/disorders/sx60.htm
Narcolepsy: Symptoms
Symptoms required for diagnosis of narcolepsy.

http://www-med.Stanford.edu/school/Psychiatry/narcolepsy/
Stanford University Center for Narcolepsy
Palo Alto, California
Under the direction of Drs. Mignot and Dement, this Stanford Center is the world leader in the search for the cause of narcolepsy. In addition to more than 100 publications, the Center has a staff of 12 people focusing on narcolepsy. Research interests range from finding better pharmacological treatments to isolating the gene for narcolepsy. An absolute must for people studying this disorder.

iv. BREATHING-RELATED SLEEP DISORDERS

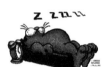

Central Sleep Apnea Informational Page

http://members.aol.com/blackcover/csa.html
Central Sleep Apnea Information Page
Discusses sleep apnea, symptoms, medical treatment, devices, etc.

http://www.newtechpub.com/phantom/
Phantom Sleep Page™ ★
Useful information about snoring and sleep apnea. References biographies, newsletters, and connections to research and support groups. Contains many links to other sites as well as S.N.O.R.E. and FAQ.

v. CIRCADIAN RHYTHM SLEEP DISORDERS

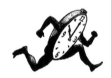

http://www.sfu.ca/~mcantle/rhythms.html
Circadian Rhythms Lab: S.F.U.
From Simon Fraser University, British Columbia, Canada, this lab is part of the psychology department. Research interests center around investigating the processes underlying nonphotic entrainment. This page exists to provide information to prospective students and colleagues in the field of circadian rhythms.

http://www.cmhc.com/disorders.sx92.htm
Circadian Rhythm Sleep Disorder
Listing of symptoms for circadian rhythm sleep disorder.

http://varesearch.ucsd.edu/klemfuss/sdsrs.html
San Diego Sleep and Rhythms Society ★
San Diego, California
A magnet for research on sleep and biological rhythms with active research programs underway at local educational institutions. Many links.

vi. OTHER SLEEP DISORDERS:

a. environmental factors. No distinct Internet references found.
b. sleep deprivation. No distinct Internet references found.
c. Restless leg syndrome

http://www.rls.org/
Restless Legs Syndrome Support Site ★
Contains listing of questions indicating whether symptoms are consistent with RLS. Offers information about RLS Foundation, subscription to Newsletter, and local support groups. Hyperlinks to recent articles, news from the medical front, and other RLS related links.

http://ourworld.compuserve.com/homepages/somno/rls.htm
Southern California Restless Legs Support Group
Presents current facts about RLS with an overview of treatments. Also offers a comprehensive review of drugs used to treat this condition. Lists support groups and letters from RLS patients. Offers information on first RLS book and contains other links to sleep disorders.

d. Nocturnal myoclonous (brief limb jerks). No distinct Internet references found.

B. Parasomnias

i. NIGHTMARE DISORDER

http://www.cmhc.com/disorders/sx48.htm
Nightmare Disorder: Symptoms
Listing of symptoms associated with nightmare disorder.

ii. SLEEP TERROR DISORDER

http://www2.micro-net.com/~dwr/
Night Terrors
Distinguishes between nightmares and night terrors. Presents symptoms and interesting facts about night terrors.

http://www.cmhc.com/disorders/sx91.htm
Sleep Terror Disorder: Symptoms
Listing of symptoms associated with sleep terror disorder.

iii. SLEEPWALKING DISORDER

http://www.cmhc.com/disorders/sx93.htm
Sleepwalking Disorder: Symptoms
Listing of symptoms associated with sleepwalking disorder.

RLSF
Restless Legs Syndrome Foundation

What is Restless Legs Syndrome?

Do you have RLS?

What is the RLS Foundation?

RLSF Information Bulletin

RLSF Medical Bulletin

Bibliography

Newsletter Subscription/Donation

Fast Facts about Night Terrors

Are not dangerous.*
Run in families.
Occur in stage 4 of the sleep cycle.
Can last 10-20 minutes.

*What you do during night terrors can be dangerous i.e walking into objects or using kitchen appliances.

C. *General Resources for Sleep~Related Disorders*

Ask A Sleep Doc

http://nshsleep.com/ask_docN.html
Ask a Sleep Doc
From Northside Hospital Sleep Disorders Center, the first accredited sleep disorders center in Georgia. Covers insomnia, sleep apnea, excessive daytime sleepiness, narcolepsy, RLS and Periodic Limb Movement Disorder, Sleepwalking, Night Terrors, Sleep Related Violence, Sleep Eating, Gastroesophageal Reflux. Mail a question to the sleep specialists and they will respond within 24 hours.

http://www.asda.org/
American Sleep Disorders Association Homepage
A professional medical association representing practitioners of sleep medicine and sleep research. Interested in diagnosis and treatment of patients with disorders of sleep and daytime alertness.

http://www.users.cloud9.net/~thorpy/LAMBERG2.HTML
Books for Sleepless Nights
List authors and quick reviews of many self-help books dealing with insomnia and related factors.

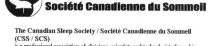

**Canadian Sleep Society
Société Canadienne du Sommeil**

The Canadian Sleep Society / Société Canadienne du Sommeil (CSS / SCS) is a professional association of clinicians, scientists and technologists formed in June 1986 to advance education and research in sleep and its disorders in Canada.

http://bisleep.medsch.ucla.edu/WFSRS/CSS/css.html
Canadian Sleep Society
Professional Association of clinicians, scientists, and technologists formed in 1986 to advance education and research on sleep and its disorders in Canada.

http://www.cmhc.com/factsfam/sleep.htm
Children's Sleep Problems
Discusses the entire range of children's sleep problems with advice to parents on how to understand and handle children who have these problems.

Shiftwork • Circadian Rhythms • Alertness • Worker Fatigue • Sleep • Shift Scheduling • Training
Work-Rest • Occupational Health & Safety • Work/Family • Fatigue Countermeasures • Human Factors
CIRCADIAN TECHNOLOGIES, INC.

Check it out...

CIRCADIAN LEARNING CENTER
Understanding Your Circadian Rhythms

Circadian Learning Center
Self-guided Tutorials on Circadian Rhythms, the Biological Clock, Alertness, and Sleep

The Shiftwork Bookstore
A Letter from the Webmaster

1998 Calendar Edition
1998 Shiftworker Family Calendars are now shipping

Round-the-Clock Child Care
Special Website Article

Website Feature
Shiftwork Poses Risk to Cardiovascular Health

NEWS BRIEFS
December 1997

Join the

Shiftwork Forum

Sign our

Guest Book

Publications new
The World's Largest Shiftwork Bookstore with Newsletters, Books, Booklets, Pamphlets, Calendar, Video – plus nearly 150 Books from *Amazon.com*.

Consulting
Shiftwork Scheduling, Lifestyle Training, Management Seminars

Research
Sleep and Alertness, Shiftwork Research, Circadian Rhythms

About Us
What is Circadian Technologies, Inc.?

http://www.circadian.com/hometext.htm
Circadian Technologies
Discusses shiftwork, circadian rhythms, alertness, and worker fatigue. Offers information on newsletters, periodicals, pamphlets, booklets and videos.

http://www.users.cloud9.net/~thorpy/NARCO.HTML
Cure Narcolepsy Now!
Facilitates communication between researchers for exchange of information leading to appropriate research in order to find the gene responsible for narcolepsy.

http://www.geocities.com/HotSprings/
1123/dsps.html
Delayed Sleep Phase Syndrome
Information on symptoms, causes, help, treatment, FAQ, and hyperlinks.

http://www.nhlbi.nih.gov/nhlbi/sleep/gp/insomnia.htm
Facts About Insomnia
Four-page brochure discussing insomnia and treatments.

http://olias.arc.nasa.gov/zteam/fredi/asdc.html
Fatigue Resource Directory: Accredited Sleep Disorders Centers
A roster of American Sleep Disorders Association Accredited Member Centers and Laboratories. Member centers provide for the diagnosis and treatment of all types of sleep-related disorders. Member laboratories specialize only in sleep-related breathing disorders.

http://www.blacksci.co.uk/products/journals/jsr.htm
Journal of Sleep Research
Lists journals by subject and title. Hyperlinks to relevant sites.

http://www.islandnet.com/~sreid/laser.html
Laser Surgery for Snoring and Sleep Apnea
Article from 1996 *Journal of Otolaryngology* discussing snoring, its cause, and the use of laser surgery as a surgical alternative.

http://smart-choice.simplenet.com/somniset.htm
Melatonin for Insomnia and Sleep Disorders
Article by Life Plus who manufacture nutritional supplements. Describes what melatonin can do. Contains a testimony page.

http://www.n-s-n.com/
National Sleep Network
Dallas, Texas

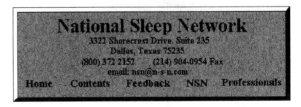

Networks sleep medicine practices and labs countrywide to provide reasonably priced access to information and tools.

http://www.ncieeg.com/
Network Concepts, Inc.
Neurology products, including digital EEG and Digital Imaging products for EEG, epilepsy monitoring, and sleep analysis.

gopher://gan.ncc.go.jp:70/0/CNET/All_files/304282
Relation of Sleep Disorders and Cancer
Information for physicians and other health care professionals published by the National Cancer Institute and discussing sleep disorders.

http://www.pslgroup.com/dg/288a2.htm

Serzone Superior in Increasing Sleep Quality

From the *Doctor's Guide to Medical and Other News*, discusses a study indicating that Serzone is associated with greater improvement of sleep quality.

http://www2.micro-net.com/~dwr/html/disorder_test.html

Sleep Disorder Test

Ten-item test to diagnose possible sleep disorders.

http://adhostnt.adhost.com/cgi-win/athealth32.exe?33

Sleep Disorders

Good discussion of the two major kinds of sleep disorders.

http://text.nlm.nih.gov/nih/cdc/www/78txt.html

Sleep Disorders of Older People

A lengthy paper from the National Institutes of Health Consensus Development Conference Statement. Discusses the findings of a panel concluding that, although sleep patterns change during the aging process, most older people with sleep disturbances suffer from a variety of medical and psychosocial disorders. Evaluations for usefulness of therapy should be made.

http://bisleep.medsch.ucla.edu/

Sleep Home Pages ★

A comprehensive resource for those involved in research or treatment of sleep or sleep-related disorders. Includes support organizations, forums, international directory of sleep researchers and physicians, etc.

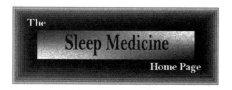

http://www.cloud9.net/~thorpy

Sleep Medicine Homepage ★★

Lists resources regarding all aspects of sleeping, including physiology, clinical sleep medicine, sleep research, federal and state information, patient information, and business-related groups. A computerized textbook of sleep medicine.

http://www.sleepnet.com/links.htm

Sleep Net's Sleep Link Reviews ★

Comprehensive listing of almost anything related to sleep. A must for anyone working in the field!

http://bisleep.medsch.ucla.edu/SRS/srs_main.htm

Sleep Research Society

Exists to promote understanding of processes of sleep and disorders through research, training and dissemination of information to scientific and medical communities.

http://www.simmonsco.com/sleep.info/sleeptest.html

Sleep Test ★

On-line scoring of a 46-item sleep test. Links to other sleep-related sites.

http://nshsleep.com/howwell.html
Sleep Test Questionnaire
Self-scoring test to help recognize symptoms of sleep disorders. Should not be used for diagnosis or treatment.

http://www.srbr.org/
Society for Research on Biological Rhythms
University of Virginia
Established in 1987, the Society attempts to promote advancement of basic and applied research in all aspects of biological rhythms.

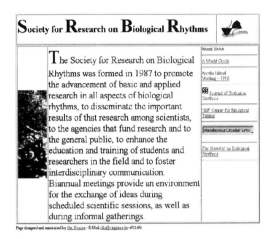

http://sids-network.org/
Sudden Infant Death Syndrome
Ledyard, Connecticut
A collaborative efforts of individuals from across the U.S. and around the world, this site offers up-to-date information as well as support for those who have been touched by the tragedy of SIDS/OID.

**Sudden Infant Death Syndrome
and Other Infant Death**

(SIDS/OID)

Information Web Site

http://www.hooked.net/~tompace/tomheadr.htm
Tom's Sleeper Page
Lists items related to sleep disorders medicine, current job listings for sleep workers, and a global listing of e-mail addresses for sleep professionals.

http://www.websciences.org/newsletter/
World Federation of Sleep Research Society
Newsletter Online
Contains hyperlinks to all articles from a worldwide perspective. References research, meetings, conference reports, historical perspectives, etc.

http://www.hep.umn.edu/~tpi-web/YAWN/YAWN.html
Young Americans with Narcolepsy
Minneapolis, Minnesota
Specializing in helping people under 30 who are recently diagnosed with narcolepsy. Contains hyperlinks, National narcolespsy registry, FAQ, supporting organizations and cover of newsletter.

Y.A.W.N.
Young Americans With Narcolepsy

A Youth Outreach and Development Organization

D. *Mailing List*

Sleep Technology Forum
listserv@dartmouth.edu
SUBSCRIBE SLPTECH Your Name

Impulse Control Disorders Not Elsewhere Classified

The essential feature of these disorders is the failure to resist an impulse, drive, or temptation to perform an act that is harmful to the person or others.

A. Intermittent Explosive Disorder, characterized by failure to resist aggressive impulses resulting in serious assaults or destruction of property.
B. Kleptomania, characterized by recurrent failure to resist impulses to steal objects not necessary for personal use or monetary value.
C. Pryomania, characterized by a pattern of fire setting for pleasure, gratification, or relief of tension.
D. Pathological Gambling, characterized by recurrent and persistent maladaptive gambling behavior.
E. Trichotillomania, characterized by recurrent pulling out of one's hair for pleasure, gratification, or relief of tension.

A. *Intermittent Explosive Disorder*

http://www.cmhc.com/disorders/sx51.htm
Intermittent Explosive Disorder: Symptoms
Brief description of symptoms of intermittent explosive disorder.

http://he.net/~bwtc/library/explosiv.html
Treating Intermittent Explosive Disorder with Neurofeedback
Case study of neurofeedback treatment.

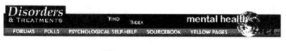

Kleptomania

SYMPTOMS

B. *Kleptomania*

http://www.cmhc.com/disorders/sx23.htm
Kleptomania: Symptoms
Brief description of symptoms of kleptomania.

C. *Pyromania*

http://www.ozemail.com.au/~jsjp/pyro.htm
Pyromania
> Article by John Hamling indicating that pathological firesetters are not a homogenous group. Hamling uses Freud's psychosexual stages as a means of subgrouping these people. The major groups are (1) oral-stage firesetters and (2) phallic stage firesetters. Treatments for each of these are discussed.

http://www.cmhc.com/disorders/sx88.htm
Pyromania: Symptoms
> Brief description of symptoms of pyromania.

D. *Pathological Gambling*

http://www.cfcg.on.ca/
Canadian Foundation on Compulsive Gambling
Willowdale, Ontario, Canada

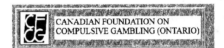

> Strives to assist those people who experience problems as a result of problem and compulsive gambling. Accomplishes this by education, treatment, research, and prevention.

http://www.gamblersanonymous.org/
Gamblers Anonymous Official Homepage
Los Angeles, California
> Contains Q & A; recovery program; phone contacts; referrals to Gam-Anon

http://www.cmhc.com/disorders/sx62.htm
Pathological Gambling, Symptoms
> *DSM-IV* symptoms.

http://www.voicenet.com/~blowry/debt.html
USA Recovery from Debt Home Page
> Offers general resources for getting out of debt including a twelve-step program. Also Christian resources for handling this problem.

E. *Trichotillomania*

http://www.tundra.org/~nannette/trich/
Resources for Trichotillomania
> Cites learning centers; bibliographies; Internet resources and other information for members of the Trichotillomania Tele-Mailer (TTM mailing list). Very informative.

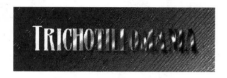

TRICHOTILLOMANIA
Compulsive Hair Pulling

Why haven't I heard of trichotillomania before?
What is trichotillomania?
What are the symptoms?
How and when does it get started?
What about infants and toddlers who pull their hair?
Does trichotillomania lead to other problems?
What is the cause?
Is it related to other illnesses?
What treatments are available?

http://www.fairlite.com/trich/
Trichotillomania
DSM-IV definition, medical information, and bulletin board.

http://www.pressenter.com/~cnovakmd/genp2.htm#B
Trichotillomania
Pioneer Clinic, St. Paul, Minnesota
Discusses trichotillomania, symptoms, how and when it gets started, infants and toddlers, cause, treatments, etc.

http://indy.radiology.uiowa.edu/Patients/IHB/Psych/Tricho.html
Trichotillomania
University of Iowa College of Medicine
Gary Gaffney discusses diagnostic features; specific culture, age and gender features; prevalence; course; differential diagnosis; comorbid conditions; treatment. Discusses medicine for trichotillomania.

F. *Mailing List*

Trichotillomania
majordomo@cs.colombia.edu
SUB TTM

Adjustment Disorders

An Adjustment Disorder is the development of a clinically significant emotional or behavioral symptom in response to an identifiable psychosocial stressor or stressors.

http://adhostnt.adhost.com/cgi-win/athealth32.exe?2

Adjustment Disorder

    Discusses the six major adjustment disorders and the characteristics associated with each. Links to causes and therapy.

http://www.mentalhealth.com/dis1/p21-aj01.html

Adjustment Disorder: American Description

    DSM-IV diagnostic criteria and associated features

http://www.mentalhealth.com/dis-rs2/p25-aj01.html

Adjustment Disorder: Research regarding Treatment

    Summaries of research studies dealing with adjustment disorders.

http://www.mentalhealth.com/rx/p23-aj01.html

Adjustment Disorder: Treatment

    Discusses medical and psychosocial treatments for adjustment disorder.

http://www.cmhc.com/disorders/sx6t.htm#psych

Adjustment Disorders: Treatment

    Discusses treatment of adjustment disorders through psychotherapy, medications, and self-help.

Adjustment Disorder   HE@LTH. At Health, Inc.

Adjustment Disorder   **Treatment**   INTERNET Mental Health

SECTION XVI.
Personality Disorders

A Personality Disorder is an enduring pattern of inner experience and behavior that deviates markedly from the expectations of the individual's culture, is pervasive and inflexible, has an onset in adolescence or early adulthood, is stable over time, and leads to distress or impairment. Personality disorders are generally divided into three clusters, based on descriptive similarities.

A. Individuals who appear odd or eccentric
i. Paranoid Personality Disorder. A pattern of distrust and suspiciousness such that others' motives are interpreted as malevolent.
ii. Schizoid Personality Disorder. A pattern of detachment from social relationships and a restricted range of emotional expression.
iii. Schizotypal Personality Disorder. A pattern of acute discomfort in close relationships, cognitive or perceptual distortions, and eccentricities of behavior.

B. Individuals who often appear dramatic, emotional, or erratic
i. Antisocial Personality Disorder. A pattern of disregard for, and violation of, the rights of others.
ii. Borderline Personality Disorder. A pattern of instability in interpersonal relationships, self-image, affects, and marked impulsivity.
iii. Histrionic Personality Disorder. A pattern of excessive emotionality and attention-seeking.
iv. Narcissistic Personality Disorder. A pattern of grandiosity, need for admiration, and lack of empathy.

C. Individuals who appear anxious or fearful
I. Avoidant Personality Disorder. A pattern of social inhibition, feelings of inadequacy, and hypersensitivity to negative evaluation.
ii. Dependent Personality Disorder. A pattern of submissive and clinging behavior related to an excessive need to be taken care of.
iii. Obsessive-Compulsive Personality Disorder. A pattern of preoccupation with orderliness, perfectionism, and control.

A. *Individuals Who Appear Odd or Eccentric*

i. *PARANOID PERSONALITY DISORDER*

http://www.mentalhealth.com/dis1/p21-pe01.html
Paranoid Personality Disorder: American Description
> *DSM-IV* diagnostic criteria, associated features, and differential diagnosis.

http://www.mentalhealth.com/dx/dx-pe01.html
Paranoid Personality Disorder: Online Diagnosis
> Quick online diagnosis for individuals or therapists. Does not substitute for clinical judgment of mental health professional.

http://www.mentalhealth.com/dis-rsl/p24-pe01.html
Paranoid Personality Disorder: Research
> Summaries of research articles dealing with paranoid personality disorder

http://www.mentalhealth.com/rx/p23-pe01.html
Paranoid Personality Disorder: Treatment
> Medical and psychosocial treatment modalities for paranoid personality disorder

Paranoid Personality Disorder
Treatment

ii. *SCHIZOID PERSONALITY DISORDER*

http://www.mentalhealth.com/dis1/p21-pe02.html
Schizoid Personality Disorder: American Description
> *DSM-IV* diagnostic criteria, associated features, and differential diagnosis.

http://www.mentalhealth.com/icd/p22-pe02.html
Schizoid Personality Disorder: European Description
> The ICD-10 Classification of Mental and Behavioral Disorders, Schizoid Personality Disorder. Presented by the World Health Organization, 1992.

http://www.mentalhealth.com/dx/dx-pe02.html
Schizoid Personality Disorder: Online Diagnosis
> Quick online diagnosis for individuals or therapists. Does not substitute for clinical judgment of mental health professional.

http://www.mentalhealth.com/dis-rsl/p24-pe02.html
Schizoid Personality Disorder: Research
> Summaries of research articles dealing with schizoid personality disorders.

Schizoid Personality Disorder
Research

http://www.mentalhealth.com/rx/p23-pe02.html
Schizoid Personality Disorder: Treatment
> Medical and psychosocial treatment modalities for schizoid personality disorder.

iii. SCHIZOTYPAL PERSONALITY DISORDER

http://www.healthguide.com/personality/schizotypal.htm
Schizotypal Personality Disorder
Offers description of and treatment for schizotypal personality disorder.

http://www.mentalhealth.com/dis-rs2/p25-pe03.html
Schizotypal Personality Disorder: Research regarding Treatment
Summary of research articles dealing with treatment of schizotypal personality disorder.

B. Individuals Who Often Appear Dramatic, Emotional or Erratic

i. ANTISOCIAL PERSONALITY DISORDER

http://www.mentalhealth.com/dis1/p21-pe04.html
Antisocial Personality Disorder: American Description
DSM-IV diagnostic criteria, associated features, and differential diagnosis.

http://www.mentalhealth.com/dis-rs3/p26-pe04.html
Antisocial Personality Disorder: Research regarding Cause
Comprehensive summaries of research articles dealing with the causes of antisocial personality disorder

http://www.mentalhealth.com/dis-rs1/p24-pe04.html
Antisocial Personality Disorder: Research regarding Diagnosis
Comprehensive summary of research articles dealing with the diagnosis of antisocial personality disorders

http://www.mentalhealth.com/dis-rs2/p25-pe04.html
Antisocial Personality Disorder: Research regarding Treatment
Comprehensive summaries of research articles dealing with the treatment of antisocial personality disorders

http://www.mentalhealth.com/rx/p23-pe04.html
Antisocial Personality Disorder: Treatment
Medical and psychosocial treatments for antisocial personality disorder

ii. BORDERLINE PERSONALITY DISORDER

BPD CENTRAL

http://members.aol.com/BPDCentral/index.html
BPD Central
A collection of resources for people interested in borderline personality disorder.

http://www.palace.net/~llama/psych/bpd.html
Borderline Personality Disorder
> Very informative regarding the causes, various approaches, psychiatric theories, and approaches used to understand one of the most controversial diagnoses in psychology today.

http://www.mentalhealth.com/dis1/p21-pe05.html
Borderline Personality Disorder: American Description
> *DSM-IV* diagnostic criteria, associated features, and differential diagnosis.

http://www.mentalhealth.com/dx/dx-pe05.html
Borderline Personality Disorder: Online Diagnosis
> Quick online diagnosis for individuals or therapists. Does not substitute for clinical judgment for mental health professional.

http://www.mentalhealth.com/rx/p23-pe05.html
Borderline Personality Disorder: Treatment
> Medical and psychosocial treatment modalities for borderline personality disorder

http://members.aol.com/BPDCentral/std_resource.html
Non-Cyberspace BPD Resources
Books dealing with BPD that can be ordered online. Contains reviews by readers.

iii. HISTRIONIC PERSONALITY DISORDER

http://www.mentalhealth.com/dis1/p21-pe06.html
Histrionic Personality Disorder: American Description
> *DSM-IV* diagnostic criteria, associated features, and differential diagnosis.

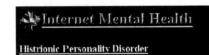

http://www.mentalhealth.com/dx/dx-pe06.html
Histrionic Personality Disorder: Online Diagnosis
> Quick online diagnosis for individuals or therapists. Does not substitute for clinical judgment of mental health professional.

http://www.mentalhealth.com/dis-rs1/p24-pe06.html
Histrionic Personality Disorder: Research
> Summaries of research articles dealing with histrionic personality disorder.

http://www.mentalhealth.com/rx/p23-pe06.html
Histrionic Personality Disorder: Treatment
> Medical and psychosocial treatment modalities for histrionic personality disorder.

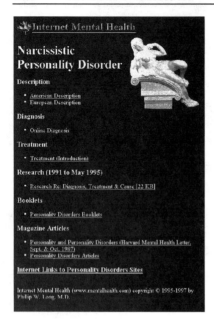

iv. NARCISSISTIC PERSONALITY DISORDER

http://www.mentalhealth.com/dis1/p21-pe07.html
Narcissistic Personality Disorder: American Description
   DSM-IV diagnostic criteria, associated features, and differential diagnosis.

http://www.mentalhealth.com/dx/dx-pe07.html
Narcissistic Personality Disorder: Online Diagnosis
   Quick online diagnosis for individuals or therapists. Does not substitute for clinical judgment of mental health professional.

http://www.mentalhealth.com/rx/p23-pe07.html
Narcissistic Personality Disorder: Treatment
   Medical and psychosocial treatment modalities for narcissistic personality disorder.

C. *Individuals Who Appear Anxious or Fearful*

i. AVOIDANT PERSONALITY DISORDER

http://www.mentalhealth.com/dis1/p21-pe08.html
Avoidant Personality Disorder: American Description
   DSM-IV diagnostic criteria, associated features, and differential diagnosis.

http://www.mentalhealth.com/dx/dx-pe08.html
Avoidant Personality Disorder: Online Diagnosis
   Quick online diagnosis for individuals or therapists. Does not substitute for clinical judgment of mental health professional.

http://www.mentalhealth.com/dis-rs1/p24-pe08.html
Avoidant Personality Disorder: Research
   Summary of research articles dealing with avoidant personality disorder.

http://www.mentalhealth.com/rx/p23-pe08.html
Avoidant Personality Disorder: Treatment
   Medical and psychosocial treatment modalities for avoidant personality disorder.

ii. DEPENDENT PERSONALITY DISORDER

http://www.mentalhealth.com/dis1/p21-pe09.html
Dependent Personality Disorder: American Description
   DSM-IV diagnostic criteria, associated features, and differential diagnosis.

http://www.mentalhealth.com/dx/dx-pe09.html
Dependent Personality Disorder: Online Diagnosis
Quick online diagnosis for individuals or therapists. Does not substitute for clinical judgment of mental health professional.

http://www.mentalhealth.com/dis-rsl/p24-pe09.html
Dependent Personality Disorder: Research
DSM-IV diagnostic criteria, associated features, and differential diagnosis.

http://www.mentalhealth.com/rx/p23-pe09.html
Dependent Personality Disorder: Treatment
Medical and psychosocial treatment modalities for dependent personality disorder.

iii. OBSESSIVE-COMPULSIVE PERSONALITY DISORDER

http://www.healthguide.com/personality/obsessive-compulsive.stm
Obsessive-Compulsive Personality Disorder
Offers description and treatment for obsessive-compulsive personality disorder.

D. Miscellaneous Resources for Personality Disorders

http://www.mhsource.com/edu/psytimes/p960241.html
Cognitive Therapy for Personality Disorders
Presents cognitive therapy as a structured, educational, and active approach to teaching patients how to identify and modify distorted thinking and dysfunctional behavior.

http://www.dlnetwork.com/millon.htm
Contemporary Trends in Assessment and Treatment of PD ★
A home study videocassette by Theodore Millon describing theoretical principles concerning personality and its development from the behavioral, cognitive, intrapsychic, and evolutionary points of view. Millon relates these to the DSM IV.

Contemporary Trends in the Assessment and Treatment of the Personality Disorders: Developments in the DSM-IV

Theodore Millon, Ph.D., University of Miami (FL)
Harvard School of Medicine (Visiting)

http:www.med.nyu.edu/Psych/screens/pds.html
Online Screening for Personality Disorders
Simple questionnaire to help determine personality traits to assist in diagnosis.

http://www.mentalhealth.com/mag1/p5h-per1.html
Personality and Personality Disorder
> Defines personality disorders; diagnosis; roots of personality; nature vs. nuture; psychoanalytic approaches; treatment; drug therapy; further readings.

Personality Disorders

This site describes the causes, symptoms, prevalence, and treatment of personality disorders. If you haven't already, please take a moment and review our **user agreement** before viewing this site.

http://www.healthguide.com/personality
Personality Disorders ★
> Describes causes, symptoms, prevalence, and treatment of personality disorders. Many good hyperlinks.

E. *Mailing Lists*

Aggression
listserv@maelstrom.stjohns.edu
SUBSCRIBE AGGRESS

Borderline Personality Disorder Support Group
listserv@maelstrom.stjohns.edu
SUBSCRIBE BORDERPD

Egoism and Antisocial
listserv@maelstrom.stjohns.edu
SUBSCRIBE EGOISM Your Name

Other Conditions That May Be a Focus of Clinical Attention

The *DSM-IV* suggests several conditions that may be a focus of clinical attention. Among those areas to be given further consideration are:

A. Medication-Induced Movement Disorders. Some disorders are included because of their importance in (1) the management of medication of mental disorders or general medical conditions, and (2) the differential diagnosis with Axis I disorders.

B. Abuse and Neglect Problems. Severe mistreatment of an individual through physical abuse, sexual abuse, or child neglect.

C. Relational Problems. Pattern of interaction resulting in significant impairment in functioning.

D. Bereavement. Adverse reaction to the death of a loved one.

A. *Medication-Induced Movement Disorders*

http://www.schizophrenia.com/ami/meds/sidefx.html
Neuroleptic-Malignant Syndrome
Describes the serious side effects of antipsychotic drugs. Discusses incidence, occurrence, mortality rate, etc.

http://www.autism.org/tardiv.html
Tardive Dyskinesia
Brief article describing symptoms, medications, and non-medication treatments for tardive dyskinesia.

B. *Abuse and Neglect Problems*

http://www.famvi.com/
Domestic Violence, Family Violence, Child Abuse Page ★
Devoted to fighting all forms of family violence and to providing information about services that are available to families in need of assistance. Links to other sites.

famvi.com

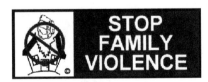

http://www.cs.utk.edu/~bartley/other/ISA.html
Incest Survivors Anonymous
An international self-help, mutual-help recovery program for men, women, and teens. ISA is run for and by survivors and their personal prosurvivors.

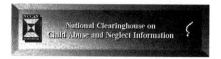

http://www.calib.com/nccanch/
National Clearinghouse on Child Abuse and Neglect ★
Washington, D.C.

> A national resource for professionals seeking information on the prevention, identification, and treatment of child abuse and neglect.

http://www.childabuse.org/
National Committee to Prevent Child Abuse ★
Chicago, Illinois

> Founded in 1972 NCPCA is a non-profit, volunteer-based organization committed to preventing child abuse in all its forms through education, research, public awareness, and advocacy.

SafetyNet

Domestic Violence Resources

http://www.cybergrrl.com/planet/dv/
Safety Net Domestic Violence Resources ★

> Contains links to areas of domestic violence projects and organizations.

C. *Relational Problems*

http://www.access.digex.net/~vqi/BirthQuest/birthqst.htm
BirthQuest!

> Online international database dedicated to searching adoptees, birth parents, adoptive parents, and siblings.

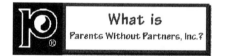

http://www.parentsplace.com/readroom/pwp/whatis.html
Parents Without Partners
Chicago, Illinois

> Founded in 1957, PWP provides single parents and their children an opportunity for enhancing personal growth, self-confidence and sensitivity toward others by offering an environment for support, friendship, and the exchange of parenting techniques.

The Sibling Support Project

http://www.chmc.org/departmt/sibsupp/
Sibling Support Project
Children's Hospital and Medical Center, Seattle, Washington

> A national program dedicated to the interests of brothers and sisters of people with special health and developmental needs.

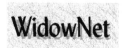

http://www.fortnet.org/WidowNet
WidowNet ★

> Information and self-help resource for, and by, widows and widowers.

http://www.wwme.org/
Worldwide Marriage Encounter
San Bernardino, California
> A weekend program offering married couples an opportunity to learn a technique of loving communication which they can use for the rest of their lives. Emphasis is on communication.

D. *Bereavement*

http://www.cmhc.com/disorders/sx39.htm
Bereavement: Symptoms
> Explains how this category can be used when the focus of clinical attention is a reaction to the death of a loved one.

http://ube.ubalt.edu/www/bereavement/
Bereavement and Hospice Support Netline ★
> An online directory of bereavement support groups and services and hospice bereavement programs across the U.S. Links to bereavement newsletters and professional associations in the grief and loss field.

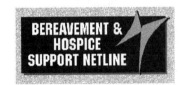

http://rivendell.org/
GriefNet ★
Ann Arbor, Michigan
> A collection of resources for those who are experiencing loss and grief. GriefNet can connect to a variety of resources related to death, dying, bereavement, and major emotional and physical losses.

GriefNet, a collection of resources of value to those who are experiencing loss and grief, is sponsored by Rivendell Resources, a non-profit foundation based in Ann Arbor, MI. This web site is mirrored in Europe by GriefNet UK. In some cases speed of access may improve if you switch sites by clicking here or on the GriefNet logo.

This web site is is best viewed with Netscape 3 (or better) or Microsoft Explorer 3.

You can SEARCH our web site here

We welcome all comments - please sign our Guest Book

About GriefNet
Help Wanted
Support Groups
Library
Bulletin Board
Bookstore
Emergency Room
Resources
Memorial Garden

http://www.sena.org/sena.html
Sena Foundation
Fredericksburg, Virginia
> A leader in the field of grief and loss for over a decade, this foundation offers free support for those going through catastrophic loss. Also offers support to those suffering loss issues resulting from aging, divorce, drug abuse, rape, and other social problems not commonly associated with grief and loss.

http://www.smartlink.net/~tag/index.html
Teen Age Grief
> A non-profit organization that provides expertise in providing grief support to bereaved teens. TAG professionals train school personnel, health professionals, law enforcement personnel, and organizations serving "at risk" youth.

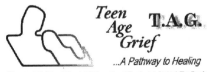

News and Updates | Events | Information | Products | Links | Feedback

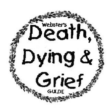

http://www.katsden.com/death/index.html
Webster's Death, Dying and Grief Resources ★
Comprehensive collection of Internet resources with a holistic perspective. Geared towards viewing death as a natural phenomenon for all people.

E. *Mailing Lists*

Partners of Abuse Survivors
listserv@maelstrom.stjohns.edu
SUBSCRIBE ABPART-L

Child Sex Abuse Witchunt
listserv@mitvma.mit.edu
SUBSCRIBE WITCHHNT

Effects of Abuse on Childbearing
reach-request@fensende.com
SUBSCRIBE

Survival (abuse survivors)
majordomo@world.std.com
SUBSCRIBE SURVIVAL

Cross Cultural Adoption Discussion
listserv@listserv.aol.com
SUBSCRIBE CCADOPTION

Facing the Death of a Loved One
listserv@maelstrom.stjohns.edu
SUBSCRIBE FACING-AHEAD

Families Coping with Illness
listserv@maelstrom.stjohns.edu
SUBSCRIBE CARINGPARENTS

Marriage and Family Therapy Counseling
    Discussion
listserv@maelstrom.stjohns.edu
SUBSCRIBE MFTC-L

Parkinson's Information Exchange
listserv@listserv.utoronto.ca
SUBSCRIBE PARKINSN

Sex Offenders Treatment
listserver@cascom.com
SUB SOPT-L Your Name

Divorce
hub@xc.org
SUBSCRIBE XN-DIVORCE

Grief, Loss, and Recovery
majordomo@listserv.prodigy.com
SUBSCRIBE GRIEF

Solutions
listserv@maelstrom.stjohns.edu
SUB SOLUTION Your Name

Child and Adolescent Anxiety and Depression
    Forum
listserv@maelstrom.stjohns.edu
SUBSCRIBE YANX-DEP

Chapter 2

Psychology/Psychiatry Search Engines

The following web sites have been specifically designed to provide links to various mental health web sites around the world. Some are more international in flavor than others. The smallest collection of links numbers a few dozen; **Mental Health Net,** listed below, has categorized over 6,000 psychology- and psychiatry-related web sites.

New sites are regularly added to most if not all of these search engines. Most but not all features from these individual sites are described below. Virtually all of the following search engines have provisions for adding individual URL's.

Visit these search engines to find psychology- and psychiatry-related sites not found in Chapter 1 and to find additional sites that relate to *DSM-IV* disorders that will be added to the World Wide Web after the publication of this edition.

<http://www.cmhc.com>
Mental Health Net ★★
CMHC Systems, Dublin, Ohio.
> CMHC provides information technology to over 500 behavioral health, public health, and human service organizations. Mental Health Net itself is a 501(c)3 not-for-profit organization. MHN now gets 30,000 hits per day.

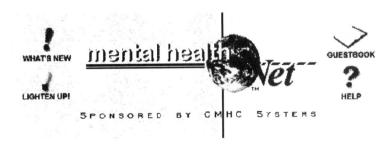

- The *Self-Help Sourcebook* lists support groups and networks throughout the world. Search by keyword or choose a problem area from a list of topics.

- *Psychological Self-Help* is an 1,000 page on-line book by Dr. Clayton E. Tucker-Ladd. Therapists may make free copies of parts of the book for their clients, and teachers may do likewise for their students. (The book is also available on floppy disk for $25.)
- The Clinician's Yellow Pages lists over 1,000 mental-health providers worldwide.
- Links to thousands of web sites that deal with the symptoms and treatment of mental disorders are listed alphabetically in the mental disorders section.
- The *Facts for Families* brochures written by the American Academy of Child and Adolescent Psychiatry are included in a special section.
- This Week in the News chronicles trends and discoveries in the field of mental health.
- Professional resources are organized alphabetically by topic. This section includes *ICD-9-CM* and *DSM* diagnostic criteria, products for sale, job links, federal and state health departments, and psychology departments. This section also mirrors Armin Guenther's Links to Psychological Journals, where over 1,000 print and electronic journals are categorized.
- The Reading Room has daily news summaries from *Join Together* and from *NewsPage* as well as press releases from the NIMH and the APA. An on-line mental-health magazine, *Perspectives*, is also published here.
- Talk to Others about current topics on the interactive discussion forums.
- Over 3,000 upcoming events are listed in the Calendar section.

Psicoenlaces Psycholinks

Ayúdanos a construir esta página enviando ^{nuevas} direcciones de interés para su inclusión en Psicoenlaces. Tambien hay disponible un directorio con clasificacion por areas geograficas.
Directorio de psicologia en Internet / Directory of psychology in Internet

<http://www.ub.es/personal/psicoen2.htm>
Psychoenlaces/Psycholinks ★★
The University of Barcelona, Spain
- Web sites can be accessed either by continent or alphabetically.
- Instructions are in English and Spanish.
- The links are an eclectic mix of URL's with a psychiatric flavor. Many sites are listed that are not found on other search engines.

<http://www.shef.ac.uk/~psysc/
psychotherapy/>

Online Dictionary of Mental Health ★★
Centre for Psychotherapeutic Studies,
University of Sheffield, England.

- Billed as Europe's largest mental
  health resource, the ODMH is
  actually international in scope.
- The Mental Health Metasearch in-
  corporates other mental health-
  related search engines, including the American Medical
  Association, the American Psychoanalytic Association, the
  China Psychological Database, the On-line Dictionary of
  Street Drug Slang, the Family Practice Handbook, Health-
  touch Drug Information, MEDline, and others. Each of these
  sites can be accessed directly by keyword.
- The Subject Index provides an alphabetical topic reference.
- Armin Guenther's *Psychological Journal Search* is mirrored
  here.
- The Library section has direct access to *Roget's Thesaurus*,
  Webster's Dictionary, the World Wide Web Virtual Library,
  The Internet Bookstore, the Online Psychology Bookstore, E-
  mail list search engines, and several medical search engines.

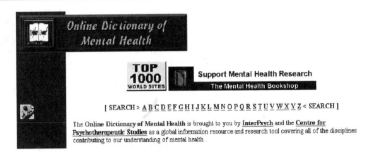

<http://mhsource.com/>

Mental Health Infosource ★★

Sponsor: CME Inc., providers of continuing education
programs

- What's New has an on-line version of *Psychiatric
  Times*, a subscription list for the MHI mailing list,
  and a collection of news articles.
- A keyword search allows the entire site to be
  accessed by individual topics.
- The Disorders and the Resources sections have
  numerous links to a wide variety of mental health
  sites.
- The Classifieds have information on practice
  opportunities, residencies and fellowships, and
  more.

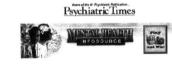

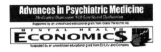

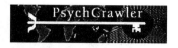

Describe what you are looking for. Click here for searching tips.

Select action. ⦿ Search on Words ⦾ Search on Concepts

Aids to refine your search: ⦿ Suggest Related Words ⦾ Suggest Alternate Spellings ⦾ Display Dictionary

Select max. number of results 25 -- then click here to

<http://www.psychcrawler.com>
Psychcrawler ★★
The American Psychological Association
- Search mental health-related topics by keyword.
- A user's guide helps visitors navigate the site.
- Psychcrawler indexes articles from the American Psychological Association, the National Insitututes of Mental Health, the Substance Abuse and Mental Health Services Administration, and the U.S. Department of Health and Human Services.

Visit the APA home page for more features at <http://www.apa.org>

The beeHive - bee's Remote Psychs

Some other good starting points are - Cognitive & Psychological Sciences on the Internet - Psych Central - Psychology links in Yahoo - Athabasca University Psychology Resources - APA - APS - CPA - Electronic Journals and Periodicals.

Here's a collection of Psychology related links taken from various places. The most recently announced are listed first. The list is long - take advantage of the "Find" button in your browser if you are looking for something specific.

<http://watarts.uwaterloo.ca/~bee/remotepsych.html>
beeHive Remote Psych Links ★★
Sponsor: Psychology Department, University of Waterloo, Ontario, Canada
- Web sites are listed chronologically on one long page; the index begins in 1995.
- Instead of just using a traditional hyperlink, the URL for each site as well as the sponsor and a brief description of each site is detailed.
- Links are provided to several other psychological search engines.

<http://www.psych-web.com/index.html>

PsychWeb ★★

The Psychology Department at Georgia Southern University in Statesboro

- Full-length web versions of *The Interpretation of Dreams* by Sigmund Freud and *Varieties of Religious Experience* by William James.
- Brochures and articles related to psychology.
- Commercial psychology sites (fee-based products and information).
- Discussion pages for college-level psychology courses.
- Find Anything allows visitors to find e-mail addresses, telephone numbers, etc.
- Armin Guenther's *Links to Psychological Journals* is mirrored here.
- Mark Lloyd's *Careers in Psychology Page* is hyperlinked.
- Other megalists of psychology takes visitors to other psych search engines.
- Psychology departments on the Web contains links to over 700 departments.
- Self-help resources are organized alphabetically by topic.
- Tip Sheets for psychology majors helps with curriculum planning, graduate admissions, and more.

Welcome to Psych Web!

<http://www.gen.emory.edu/medweb/medweb.mentalhealth.html>

MedWeb ★★

Atlanta Georgia's Emory University Health Sciences Center Library

- The MedWeb search engine covers all of medicine and has a fine section on mental health, psychiatry, and psychology. Over 8,000 links are now categorized.
- A keyword search allows for search by topic.
- The Country Index categorizes URL's in more than 100 countries.
- The Regions Index references URL's by continent.
- The What's New sections lists sites recently added.

MedWeb Mental Health/Psychiatry/Psychology

AIDS and HIV . Academic Departments . Academic Programs . Adolescent Psychiatry . Advice columns . Alternative medicine . Alzheimer's Disease . Anorexia . Anxiety . Art Therapy . Art therapy . Attention Deficit Disorder . Bibliographies . Bioethics . Biofeedback . Biography . Biology . Biomathematics and biostatistics . Bipolar Disorders . Classification . Clinical Practice . Companies . Conferences and Calendars . Consumer health . Continuing education . Databases . Deafness . Dementia . Depression . Developmental Disabilities . Directories . Disabilities . Disasters . Discussion groups . Diseases . Documents . Down's Syndrome . Eating Disorders . Education . Educational resources . Electronic Documents . Electronic publications . Emergency medicine . Endocrinology . Environment . Family medicine . Frequently asked questions . Genetics and molecular biology . Geriatrics . Guidelines . Guides . Gynecology and women's health . Health Psychology . Health care policy . History . Hospitals . Hypnosis . Indices . Informatics . Institutes and agencies . Internal Medicine . Legal Medicine . Legal medicine . Lists of Internet Resources . Medical Education . Medical Illustration . Medical Libraries . Medical Products . Memory . Mental Retardation . Military Medicine . Neurology . Neurosciences . Neurosurgery . News . Nursing . Nutrition . Occupational Therapy . Oncology . Online Addiction . Panic Disorder . Patient education . Pediatrics . Pharmacy and Pharmacology . Physical Medicine and Rehabilitation . Post Traumatic Stress Disorders . Preventive Medicine . Projects . Psychopharmacology . Psychophysiology . Public Health . Publishing . Rehabilitation . Religion and Medicine . Residencies . Review Literature . Schizophrenia . Self-help groups . Services . Sexual abuse . Sites . Sleep . Social Work . Societies and associations . Software . Substance Dependence . Suicide . Support Groups . Terminology . Travel Medicine . Veterinary Medicine . Virtual reality in medicine . Wit and Humor . schizophrenia

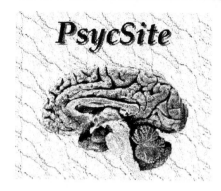

<http://stange.simplenet.com/psycsite/>

PsycSite ★★

Sponsor: Nipissing University in Ontario, Canada

Features:

- How to Use These Resources guides visitors through this extensive site.
- Info Sources for Psychology has pointers to journals, abstracts, and databases.
- Other Psychology Launch Pads has links to general psychology sites.
- List Servers and News Groups is a listing of list servers and news groups dealing with psychology.
- Psychology Related Software has downloadable shareware and commercial products.
- University Connections has a listing of universities and links to several other departments.
- Professional Centre lists professional organizations and societies plus conference information.
- Student Centre has information on grad schools and other helpful hints.
- Resource Persons has addresses of volunteers with expertise in various areas.
- Chat Room is a place where visitors can talk to each other.
- Research Centre conducts on-line psychological studies.

Non Mainstream Psychotherapy and Counselling Resources on the Internet

<http://psyctc.sghms.ac.uk/mirrors/non-main/nonmain.htm>

Non-Mainstream Psychotherapy and Counselling Resources on the Internet ★★

Nick Totton

- Therapies section is divided into body-oriented therapies, expressive therapies, spiritually-oriented therapies, psychodynamic therapies, and humanistic, growth movement and process therapies.
- Resources lists alternative and general web sites in alphabetical order.
- Practitioners lists directories and individual therapists with a holistic approach.
- New Models and Paradigms lists different orientations to the discipline.
- Organizations is a brief list of ecclectic groups and societies.

<http://www.healthatoz.com/>
HealthAtoZ ★
Medical Network, Inc.
- HealthAtoZ has 27 health-related search engines including one on mental health with several hundred links.
- Topics may be searched by keyword.
- Mental Health topics are divided into nine areas:
  Alternative Therapies
  Advocacy and Support Groups
  Diseases and Conditions
  Institutes and Organizations
  Journals and Periodicals
  Mailing Lists
  Newsgroups
  Psychology, and
  Products and Services
- Listed sites are rated and reviewed.

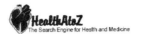
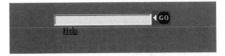

Mental Health

* Advocacy & Support Groups (136)
* Alternative Therapies (33)
* Diseases and Conditions (250)
* Institutes & Organizations (25)
* Journals and Periodicals (10)
* Mailing List (5)
* NewsGroups (1)
* Psychology (97)
* Products and Services (46)

<http://www.mentalhealth.org/>
Knowledge Exchange Network (KEN) ★★
From U.S. National Mental Health Services, part of the U.S. Department of Health and Human Services.
- Mental Health Links are organized by topic.
- Mental Health Statistics are also available.
- Listed sites are thoroughly reviewed.

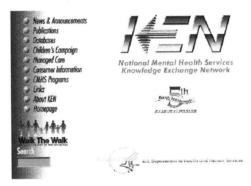

<http://www.freenet.msp.mn.us/ip/stockley/mental_health.html>
Internet Mental Health Resources ★
Herbert D. Stockley
- Resources are grouped by category.

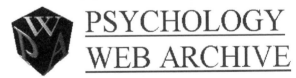

Internet Mental Health Resources

<http://swix.ch/clan/ks/CPSP1.htm>
Psychology Web Archive ★
Karsten Schwarz, University of Zurich, Switzerland
- Listed sites are in English and German.
- Many links relate to social psychology
- Sites are categorized by:
  Articles
  Abstracts and References
  Software
  Libraries and Journals
  Gopher Resources
  Searching the Web
  Social Psychology
  Clinical Psychology
  More Psychology Resources
  Miscellaneous

Jumping Off Place for Social Psychologists

PSYCHOLOGY WEB ARCHIVE

- Social Psychology
- Articles and References
- Software
- Libraries and Journals
- Gopher Resources
- Searching the Web

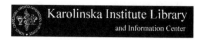

Behavioral and Mental Disorders (Non MeSH)

<http://www.mic.ki.se/Diseases/f3.html>
Behavioral and Mental Disorders ★★
The Karolinska Institute in Stockholm, Sweden
- Selected web sites focus on disorders.
- Sites listed are primarily informational and descriptive.
- Countries of origin are given for listed sites.

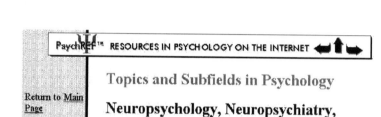

16. <http://seamonkey.ed.asu.edu/%7Egail/resource.htm>
The Counseling Web ★
Gail Hackett, Arizona
Links are organized by:
    Counseling Resources
    Mental Health Resources
    Directories of Psychological Resources
    Psychiatric and Neurosciences Resources
    Research Information on the WWW
    Resources for Educators

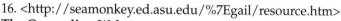

PsychREF™ RESOURCES IN PSYCHOLOGY ON THE INTERNET ⬅ ⬆ ➡

Return to Main Page

Topics and Subfields in Psychology

Neuropsychology, Neuropsychiatry, and Behavioral Neurology

<http://maple.lemoyne.edu/~hevern/psychref4-9.html#general>
Resources in Psychology on the Internet ★★
The Psychology Department at Lemoyne University, a Jesuit college in Central New York
- General Resources includes journals, professional associations and societies, and history of psychology.
- Teaching/Research/Student Resources includes general teaching, conferences, research, ethical issues, on-line courses, academic assistance, media and psychology, books and publishers online, and computer software for psychology.
- Topical Resources includes clinical psychology/psychiatry and counseling, specific clinical problems and disorders, developmental psychology, life span development, social psychology, behavioral medicine and health psychology, disabilities and rehabilitation medicine, neuropsychology and neuropsychiatry, neurological disorders, psychological testing, gay, lesbian, and bisexual resources, psychology of women, and miscellaneous.

Dr. Bob's Mental Health Links

Welcome to my page of mental health links. Its target audience is mental health professionals, but it's open to all.

If you know of something informative (or interesting) that I don't have listed, please feel free to email me to let me know.

<http://uhs.bsd.uchicago.edu/dr-bob/mental.html>
Dr. Bob's Mental Health Links ★★
Robert Hsiung, M.D.
- Dr. Bob's Virtual En-psych-lopedia includes Psychopharmacology Tips and a few general resources.
- The Comprehensive section includes other large and small search engines.
- Focused Content has an alphabetical listing of psychology- and psychiatry-related topics.
- Organizations section lists associations worldwide.
- Psychiatry Departments are hyperlinked.
- A list of other Universities is hyperlinked.
- Psychology- and Psychiatry-related Publications are listed.
- Hardware and Software section offers links to computer sites.
- Miscellaneous includes Off the Beaten Track, Partisans, Ethics, Management of Care, and General Medicine.

<http://www.mentalhealth.com>
MentalHealth.Com: Sharing Mental Health Knowledge with the World ★★
Phillip W. Long, M.D.
- An alphabetical Index allows the site to be searched by letter.
- Disorders offers information on description, diagnosis, treatment, and research findings for the 52 most common mental disorders.
- Medications includes indications, contraindications, warnings, precautions, adverse affects, overdose, dosage, and research findings for the 67 most commonly prescribed medications.
- Magazine has news, magazine articles, booklets, stories of recovery, letters, and editorials.
- Diagnosis has on-line diagnosis tests for several disorders.
- Internet Links has hyperlinks to other sites.

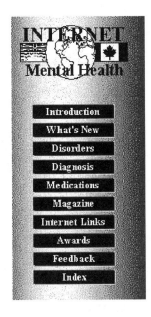

[Home | Starting Points | Directories | Journals | Associations | Conferences | Software]
[Search | Contributors | What's New]

Resources for Psychology and Cognitive Sciences on the Internet

<http://www.ke.shinshu-u.ac.jp/psych/index.html>
Resources for Psychology and Cognitive Sciences on the Internet ★
Shinsu University, Nagano, Japan
- A keyword search is available.
- Categorizations include:
  Starting Points for Psychology and Cognitive Sciences
  Directories of Psychology and Cognitive Sciences
  Electronic Journals and Papers
  Associations
  Conferences
  Software Archives and Information
  Online Bookstores
  Online Library Information
  What's New
  Comments
- An additional Announcement Section includes:
  Armin Guenther's *List of Psychological Journals*
  A Mailing List for Psychology and the Internet (in Japanese)
  Psychological Documents Archive in Japan (in Japanese)
  Archives of the Symposium on Educational Psychology and
  the Internet (in Japanese)

<http://www.sosig.ac.uk>
Social Science Information Gateway ★★
The UK Economic and Social Research Council
The Electronic Libraries Programme
The European Commission through the DESIRE Project

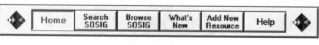

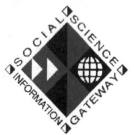

- SOSIG has links to a variety of social science sites: Economics; Education; Environmental Issues; Ethnology and Social Anthropology; Feminism; Geography, Government and Military Science; Law; Management, Accountancy, and Business; Philosophy, **Psychology**, General Social Science and Methodology; Social Welfare, Community, and Disability; Sociology; Statistics and Demography.
- SOSIG links to:
  Electronic Journals
  Reports and Papers
  Educational Software
  Electronic Newsletters

Home Pages of Social Science Organizations
Digitized Books
Scholarly Mailing Lists and Archives
Databases
Datasets
Bibliographies
- Topics can be searched by keyword.

<http://psych.hanover.edu/>
Hanover College Psychology Department ★
Hanover College, Indiana
- The Psychology Department's Home Page has categories for:
  Psychological Software
  Psychological Societies
  Publishers
  Miscellaneous Psychology Links
  Psychology Tutorials
  Electronic Journals
  Internet Searching
- Visitors may participate in on-line psychology experiments.

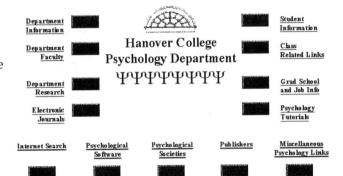

<http://www.bubl.ac.uk/> (use BUBL search features)
BUBL Link Information Service ★★
Andersonian Library, Strathclyde University, Glasgow, Scotland
- BUBL has links to many subjects including psychology, psychiatry, social psychology, artificial intelligence, and physiology and neuroscience.
- Psychology categories include:
  Psychology General Resources
  Psychology Departments
  Psychology Societies
  Psychology Journals
  Sensory Perception, Movement, Emotions, and Physiological Drives
  Conscious Mental Processes and Intelligence
  Subconscious and Altered States and Processes
  Differential and Developmental Psychology
  Applied psychology
- Psychiatry links include Diseases of the Nervous System and Mental Disorders.

BUBL Information Service

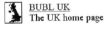

A national information service for the higher education community, funded by JISC

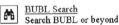 BUBL Link
The Subject Tree

BUBL Journals
Abstracts, full text, hundreds of titles

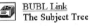 BUBL Search
Search BUBL or beyond

BUBL News
Jobs, events, surveys, updates

BUBL UK
The UK home page

BUBL Mail
Mailing lists and mail archives

BUBL Archive
LIS, journals, Internet development

BUBL Admin
About BUBL: FAQ, feedback, funding

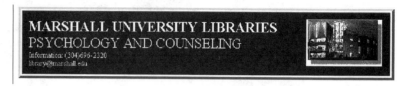

<http://www.marshall.edu/library/psylist.htm>
Psychology and Counseling on the Web ★
Marshall University Libraries, Huntington, West Virginia
- This search engine is categorized into:
  Directories (including Behavioral, Clinical, and Educational)
  Journals and Magazines
  Professional Organizations
  Online Periodical and Resource Lists
  Internet Search Tools
  Electronic Citation Style Sheets
- Sites are organized alphabetically within each category.

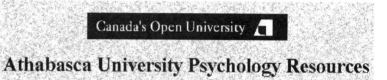

<http://server.bmod.athabascau.ca/html/aupr/psycres.htm>
Athabasca University Psychology Resources ★★
Athabasca University Psychology Centre, Athabasca, Alberta, Canada
   Categories include:
   Behavioural
   Biological
   Clinical
   Cognitive
   Demonstrations and Tutorials
   Departments of Psychology
   Developmental Psychology
   Educational Psychology
   History of Psychology
   Journals
   Psychology Megasites
   Organizational and Industrial Psychology
   Social Psychology
   Psychological Software
   Sports Psychology
   Student Resources

<http://www.psychologie.uni-bonn.de/home_e.htm>
Psychology Online ★★
Bonn University, Germany

- This site has English and German versions.
- There is a listing of Psychological Institutes worldwide.
- Psychological On-line Documents are categorized.
- A listing of past, present, and upcoming Psychological Conferences is available in English.
- WWW sites for Experimental and Cognitive Psychology are listed in English.
- WWW sites for Clinical Psychology are listed in English.

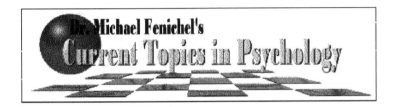

<http://www.tiac.net/biz/drmike/Current.shtml>
Current Topics in Psychology ★
Clinical psychologist Dr. Michael Fenichel

- Listing of links to articles, web sites, and research tools.
- Specific topics in psychology are listed alphabetically.

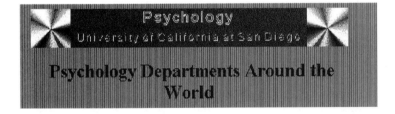

<http://psy.ucsd.edu/>
Psychology Departments Around the World ★
University of California at San Diego Psychology Department

- The Web's most extensive listing of academic Psychology Departments.
- Other Psychology-Related Sites is a mini-search engine.
- Both categories are accessed alphabetically.

<http://www.einet.net/galaxy/Social-Sciences/Psychology.html>

Galaxy: The Professional's Guide to a World of Information ★
TradeWave Corporation

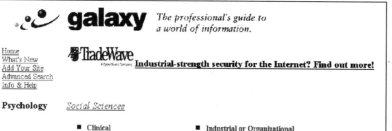

- Psychology sites are categorized by:
  Clinical
  Developmental
  Educational
  Experimental
  Industrial or Organizational
  Motivation
  Personality
  Physiological
  Social

- This site also has links under the following categories:
  Academic Organizations
  Announcements
  Books
  Collections
  Discussion Groups
  Events
  Guides
  Organizations
- Information may be searched by keyword.
- Galaxy has links to sites that cover:
  Anthropology
  Communication
  Education
  Geography
  History
  Library and Information Science
  Political Science
  Sociology

<http://www.med.umich.edu/psych>

Psychiatry Star ★
The University of Michigan Department of Psychiatry
- General References of Interest in Psychiatry are classified according to:
  Psychiatric Disorders
  Psychiatric Treatments
  Psychiatrically Oriented Institutions
  Pscchology Oriented Information Services
- The site also has a section for Medical References.

<http://alabanza.com/kabacoff/Inter-Links/health/psy/psy
.html>
Psychological Resources ★
Inter-Links by Rob Kabacoff, Ph.D.
Psychology sites are categorized by:
> Resource Collections
> Discussions (including electronic mailing lists, newsgroups
> and support newsgroups)
> Other (conferences, medication, software, testing)

<http://www.medmatrix.org/SPages/
Psychiatry.asp>
Medical Matrix ★★
Healthtel Corporation

- Medical Matrix is a medical search engine with many links relating to psychiatry, neurology, public health, and other mental health-related topics.
- Over 3,000 sites are categorized with respect to:
  Speciality and Disease Categorized Information
  Clinical Practice
  Literature
  Education
  Healthcare and Professionals
  Computers, Internet, and Technology
  Marketplace
- Topics can be searched by keyword.
- A Start Search features allows searching through:
  The Merck Manual
  Reuters Medical News
  Clinical Pharmacology (drug monographs)
  Family Practice Handbook
  The Health Explorer (patient handouts)
  PubMed Medline (peer-reviewed abstracts)

MEDICAL MATRIX
Ranked, Peer-Reviewed,
Annotated, Updated
Clinical Medicine Resources

- MEDLINE
- JOURNALS
- CME
- NEWS
- RX ASSIST
- TEXTBOOKS
- STAT SEARCH NEW!
- PATIENT EDUCATION
- MARKETPLACE

check new listings ● *suggest a new URL* ● *rate current sites*
NEW! *participate in the Medical Matrix Forums* NEW!
about Medical Matrix ● *about the Editorial Board* ● *the webmasters*

Psychiatry

News Abstracts Reviews Articles Meeting Reports Major Resources
Reference Documents Indices Learning Modules Procedures Decision Tools
Practice Guidelines Cases Meetings Textbooks Diseases CME Forums
Patient Education Marketplace

<http://fly.hiwaay.net/~garson
Magic Stream: Guide to Emotional Wellness ★
Regina P. Garson
> Magic Stream's WebDex contains references on psychology, psychiatry, and self-help with a holistic slant.

Magic Stream Journal
...a guide to emotional wellness:

Psychological information on the Web is now sizeable. Academic Psychology, the mental health disciplines, self-help and many related topics are represented in varying degrees of informativeness. We have tried to provide a wide array of links into these domains. Several indices listed below provide far more exhaustive resources.

Psychology-related Newsgroups	Psychology-related Research Specialties and Subdisciplines	Resources in Mental Health and Professional Psychology
College and University Psychology Departments	Scientific Journals in Psychology and Related Disciplines	Professional Societies in Psychology and Organizations Related to Mental Health

<http://www.albany.edu/psy/other.html#top>
Psychology Related Web and Internet Information ★★
State University of New York at Albany
> Links are categorized in the following sections:
> Psychology-related Newsgroups
> College and University Psychology Departments
> Psychology-related Research Specialties and Subdisciplines
> Scientific Journals in Psychology and Related Disciplines
> Resources in Mental Health and Professional Psychology
> Professional Societies in Psychology and Organizations Related to Mental Health

<http://www.grohol.com/>
Psych Central ★★
Dr. John Grohol

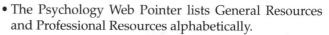

- The Psychology Web Pointer lists General Resources and Professional Resources alphabetically.
- The Mailing List Pointer lists psychology-related mailing lists alphabetically.
- The Newsgroup pointer lists newsgroups under various categories.
- Page One welcomes original articles and op-ed pieces.
- The Mental Disorder Symptom Lists covers a variety of disorders.
- The Booklist has reviews of a number of psychology-related books.
- The Suicide Helpline lists suicide resources on the Internet.

<http://netpsych.com>
NetPsych.com ★
NetPsych.com

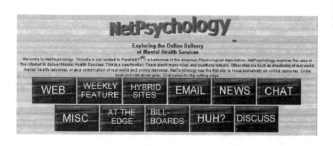

- Hybrid Sites and Web list and review an eclectic group of URL's.
- Keyword search is available.
- Several psychology-related Chat Rooms and Newsgroups are listed.
- NetPsych.com pays particular attention to the on-line delivery of services.

<http://www.med.nyu.edu/Psych/>
NYU Department of Psychiatry ★
New York University Psychiatry Department

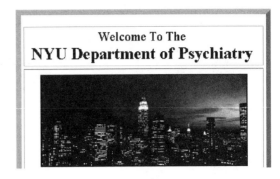

- Information for the General Public includes several On-line Screening Tests.
- The Reference Desk has links for psychologists and psychiatrists.
- Interactive Testing in Psychiatry has seven test modules with 30 board-style questions per module. Scoring is instant, and CME credit is available.
- An on-line slide show, Augmentation Strategies in the Treatment of Depression, has 41 slides containing a text version and a references list. CME credit is available.
- For Medical Students Only has several helpful student-related links.

<http://www.onlinepsych.com/>
Online Psych ★★
Online Psychological Services Inc.

- Over 7,000 print titles are available in the Online Bookstore.
- The Message Board allows visitors to interact with other visitors.
- Mental Health Info has more than 250 links alphabetized in 25 topic sections.

<http://www.umdnj.edu/psyevnts/psyjumps.html>
Meetings, Organizations, and Resources in Behavioral Healthcare ★★
Dr. Myron Pulier, Department of Psychiatry, New Jersey Medical School

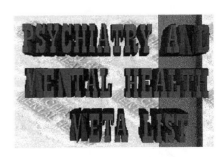

- A worldwide calendar of events and meetings for mental health professionals.
- Over 1,500 mental-health organizations are listed.
- Web resources in psychiatry are listed; many are reviewed.

<http://www2.cybernex.net/~jas/index.html>
Psychiatry and Mental Health Meta List ★
J. Steinbock, L.C.S.W.

- A direct keyword search is available to *Mental Health Net*.
- This list concentrates on linking to psychology and psychiatry search engines.

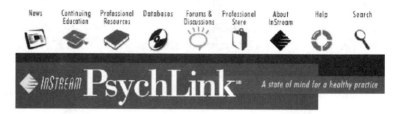

<http://www.psychlink.com/>

PsychLink ★

The InStream Corporation

- Free membership is required for access to certain categories.
- PsychLink provides up-to-date news on mental health-related topics; articles are archived and can be accessed by keyword search.
- There is information on Continuing Education and Products.
- PsychLink hosts Discussions and Forums for site members.

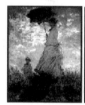

· *Specifica* ·

An evolving resource of information and services for people in need

<http://www.realtime.net/~mmjw>

Specifica ★

Jeanine Wade, Ph.D., Austin, Texas

    Mental Health Links are categorized under:

    General

    Specific Problem Areas

    General Information for Professionals

WWW Psychology Resources

MENU: General Resources | Area-specific Resources | Australian Psychology Departments | Psychology Departments World-wide | Medline, PsychINFO and PCI | Add a Link to this Page

<http://www.psy.uwa.edu.au/ptrspsy.htm#PSYCH-SPECIFIC>

WWW Psychology Resources ★★

University of Western Australia

- General Resources includes:
  Professional Bodies
  On-line Services
  Psychology-related Newsgroups and Mailing Lists
  E-Journals and Periodicals
  Psychology-related Commercial Sites
  Other
- Area Specific Resources are listed alphabetically.
- Psychology Departments worldwide are included.

<http://www.psychology.com>
Psychology.com ★
Integrated EAP Inc.
- The Psychological Testing Service lists a variety of professionally developed personality tests.
- The Therapist Directory is a geographically organized list of mental health providers.
- Cyber-Psych is the web site's mental health search engine, organized by categories.

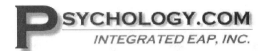

PSYCHOLOGY.COM
INTEGRATED EAP, INC.

This web site has been created to help people enhance their personal and professional lives.

- Psychological Testing Service
  Select from a variety of professionally developed personality tests.
- Therapist Directory
  A geographically organized list of psychiatrists, psychologists, and social workers.
- Employee Assistance Program
  A cost-effective benefit to help employees and their family members find solutions for a variety of adverse situations.
- Cyber-Psych
  A web link to a wealth of psychological resources

<http://www.wiso.uni-augsburg.de/sozio/hartmann/psycho/journals.html>
Links to Psychological Journals ★★
Armin Guenther, University of Augsburg, Germany
- An index of links to more than 1,000 psychology and social science journal sites ordered by journal name.
- This site is mirrored at several other sites, including:
  Mental Health Net (USA)
  PsychWeb (USA)
  Shinshu University (Japan)
  University of Sheffield (UK)
  School of Behavioural Sciences, Macquarie University (Australia)
- Full text journal editions are not available at this site; nearly all sites provide some general journal information.
- Keyword search is available.

Links to Psychological Journals

by Armin Günther, Augsburg, in cooperation with Martien Brand, Amsterdam

An Index of 1,000+ Psychology and Social Science Journals Online

Covering English, German, French, Dutch, and Spanish language journals; providing general journal information (nearly all), tables of contents (many), abstracts (some), or full text articles (few).
NEW Try our new US-mirror with added functionality! NEW

WEB RESOURCES FOR SOCIAL WORKERS

General Information | Social Work Schools | Politically Speaking

<http://www.colostate.edu/depts/SocWork/webstuff.html>
Web Resources for Social Workers ★
Colorado State University Department of Social Work
An alphabetical list of helpful links for those in the social work profession.

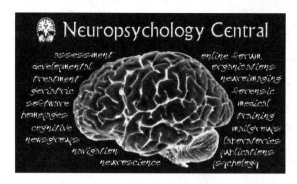

<http://www.premier.net/~cogito/neuropsy.html>
Neuropsychology Central ★★
Jeffrey Browndyke, M.A., Louisiana State University
  • The Psychology Section of this neuropsychology site has links to general psychology web sites.
  • This site is a search engine for neuropsychology topics and is also listed in Chapter Three.

A Guide to Mental Health on the Internet in Australia

<http://www.powerup.com.au/~qamh/link.html>
A Guide to Mental Health on the Internet in Australia ★
Queensland Association for Mental Health
Links are categorized by:
        Community Organisations
        Professional Associations
        Institutes and Other Projects
        University Departments
        Government Sites
        Hospitals: Public and Private
        Commercial Organisations and Private Links
        Others
        On-line Journals

JOURLIT - BOOKREV -DUALLOOK Information

<http://apsa.org/jourlit/index.htm>
Jourlit-Bookrev Bibliographic Data Search ★★
The American Psychoanalytic Association
  • Over 30,000 references, which include journal articles, book reviews, and other publications, can be accessed by keyword. The included journals are listed.
  • More advanced users can order software that allows them to print bibliographies, program user-created output, and merge results of multiple searches.
  • Reprints can be ordered by phone, fax, or e-mail.

The Australian WWW Psychiatry Resources Directory

<http://www.cundle.com.au/gen/psych/psychres.html>
Australian WWW Psychiatry Resources Directory ★
Dr. Bruce Farnsworth, Manning Base Hospital, TAREE
        The site is categorized according to:
        Australian Medical Resources
        Australian Departments of Psychiatry
        International Psychiatric Hospitals and Institutes
        World Wide Psychiatry Resources

<http://www.behavenet.com/>

BehaveNet: Behavioral Health Care Information and Publishing on the World Wide Web ★

BehaveNet—Publishing, hosting, and listing services

> Instead of providing links to psychology- or psychiatry-related information sites, BehaveNet is oriented toward the academic, administrative, and professional segments of behavioral science.

BehaveNet® Inc
Behavioral health care information & publishing on the World Wide Web since 1995

BehaveNet® Directories
Academic Centers || Advocacy Organizations || Boards of Examiners || Classified || Continuing Education || Forensic Examiners || Government Agencies || Law || Legislatures || Print Publications || Products || Providers || Professional Associations || Support Organizations || Treatment Guidelines

<http://strauss.ihs.ox.ac.uk/oxamweb.html>

OXAMWEB: Mental Health in 3 Clicks ★

National Health Service Research and Development Programme, Anglia and Oxford Region; the Medical Research Council, UK

> On-line articles, information, and links to a variety of psychology- and psychiatry-related sites.

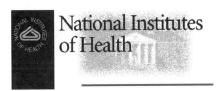

<http://www.nih.gov/>

National Institutes of Health Home Page ★★

National Institutes of Health, Bethesda, Maryland

> The NIH web site includes a search engine with references to many disorders. References are primarily informational for clinicians and clients, and hyperlinks to other web sites are not generally included.

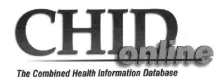

<http://chid.nih.gov/>

CHID online: the Combined Health Information Database ★★

Produced by several health-related agencies of the U.S. Federal Government

> • CHID lists a wealth of health promotion and education materials that are not indexed elsewhere.
>
> • A simple or detailed keyword search is available
>
> • Current topics are more oriented toward physical disabilities, but many mental disorders are covered, and the list of topics will constantly be expanding.

<http://www.healthfinder.gov/>

Healthfinder ★★

U.S. Department of Health and Human Services

> • Selected on-line publications, clearinghouses, databases, web sites, and support and self-help groups.
>
> • Also links to government and not-for-profit agencies that produce reliable information for the public.

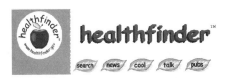

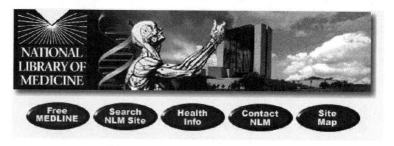

<http://www.nlm.nih.gov/>

The National Library of Medicine ★★

National Institutes of Health

- The world's largest medical library. Supports a national and international network of local and regional medical libraries.
- NLM produces MEDLINE, a computer index to over 3,800 international medical journals. MEDLINE does not contain the full text of journal articles.
- MEDLARS (MEDical Literature Analysis and Retrieval System) is a computerized system of 40 on-line databases containing about 18 million references.
- A list of NLM Fact Sheets listed alphabetically help browers navigate the system.
- NLM Locator searches the book holdings database (CATLINE), the audiovisual holdings database (AVLINE), the journal holdings database (SERLINE), and the directory of information resources (DIRLINE) of the U.S. National Library of Medicine.
- MESH is the NLM's controlled vocabulary thesaurus, with more than 18,000 main headings.
- Free searching is available through the Internet Grateful Med or PubMed search systems.

<http://www.yahoo.com/Science/Psychology>

Yahoo Psychology Section

- Yahoo is the only major all-purpose search engine that has adequately categorized mental health web sites.
- Sites are divided into:

Indices	Organizations
Companies	Parapsychology
Counseling and Therapy	Psychiatry
Disciplines	Psychologists
Education	Publications
Hypnosis	Sleep and Dreams
Libraries	Software
Mental Health	Tests and Experiments
Museums	Usenet

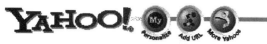

- Companies@
- Conferences (20) NEW!
- Counseling and Therapy@
- Disciplines (236) NEW!
- Education (265) NEW!
- Humor@
- Hypnosis@
- Libraries (3)
- Mental Health@
- Museums (1)
- Organizations (89)
- Parapsychology@
- Psychiatry@
- Psycholinguistics@ NEW!
- Psychologists (37)
- Publications (36)
- Sleep and Dreams (71) NEW!
- Software (5)
- Tests and Experiments (34) NEW!
- Usenet (18)

http://www.socsciresearch.com/
**Research Resources for the Social
Sciences** ★★
McGraw-Hill Ryerson
   Includes links to the following subjects:
      Psychology
      Sociology/Anthropology
      Demography
      News/Journalism
      Women's Studies
      Others

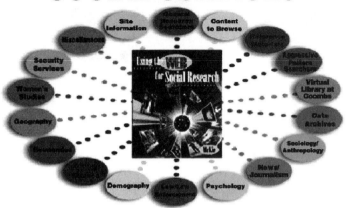

<http://www.iop.bpmf.ac.uk/home/depts/library/
psy/meta.htm>
Institute of Psychiatry Library: Mental Health ★★
Institute of Psychiatry Library, Kings College London,
University of London

 **IoP Library: Mental Health:
Lists & search engines**

   Referenced sites are categorized by:

Starting Points and Search Engines	Tourette Syndrome
Affective Disorders	Mailing Lists and Newsgroups
Attention Deficit Disorders	Anxiety Disorders
Chronic Fatigue Syndrome	Bereavement and Loss
Crime/Forensic	Communicative Disorders
Dyslexia	Disabled
Evidence-Based Mental Health	Electroencephalography
Health Policy	Family
Parapsychology	Multiple Sclerosis
Psycholinguistics	Personality
Religion and Psychology	Psychotherapy
Software	Sleep Disorders
Suicide	Substance Use Disorders
Institutions	Violence
Alzheimer's Disease	Online Journals
Autism	Art
Classification	Child Psychiatry
Dementia	Consciousness
Eating Disorders	Dissociative Disorders
Factitious Disorders	Ethics
Mental Retardation	Geriatric Psychiatry
Parkinson's Disease	Neurology/Neurosciences
Psychological Tests	Psychiatric Status Rating Scales
Schizophrenia	Psychotropic Drugs
Stress Disorders	

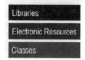 Internet Resources

Libraries
Electronic Resources
Classes

Mental Health Resources

<http://www.hsls.pitt.edu/intres/mental/mhr.html>
Mental Health Resources ★★
Health Sciences Library System, University of Pittsburgh, Pennsylvania
Resources are oganized by:
Mental Health Administration
Book Reviews
Calendar of Events/Conferences
Classification and Assessment Resources
Classifieds
Continuing Medical Education
Computer and Database Resources
Directory and Atlas Resources
Electronic Mental Health Journals and Newspapers
Government Agencies
Grants and Research
Institutions
Locating Psychological and Psychiatric Tests
Managed Health Care Resources
Nursing
Patient Education for Mental Health
Products, Services, and Software
Psychiatric Resources Arranged by Topic
Mailing Lists
Usenet Groups
Publishers
Search Engines
Statistics
University Psychiatric Departments
WPIC Library Core Journals

Chapter 3
General Sites
of Interest to Clinicians

A. *Neuropsychology*

<http://neurosurgery.mgh.harvard.edu/abta/diction.htm>
ABTA Dictionary for Brain Tumor Patients
American Brain Tumor Association

    All the terms that a patient with a brain tumor might encounter.

<http://www.aan.com/>
The American Academy of Neurology ★
St. Paul, Minnesota

- Fact sheets and brochures on a variety of neurological conditions and procedures.
- Neurology news and information.
- The Patient Information Guide has an alphabetical listing of neurology-related topics to help patients and physicians locate services.

<http://www.med.usf.edu/ASN/asn.html>
American Society for Neurochemistry
Galveston, Texas

    For investigators in the field of neurochemistry.

<http://www.tbidoc.com/>
Brain Injury and Neuropsychology ★
Antoinette Appel, Plantation, Florida

- Devoted to the understanding of brain injury.
- Includes information on testing, medication, statutory definitions, and neuro-imaging.

ABTA Dictionary for Brain Tumor Patients

This dictionary explains terms the patient with a brain tumor is likely to hear or read. For additional information, consult with the medical professionals caring for you or refer to a medical dictionary or text book.

<http://www.div40.org/>
Division 40: Clinical Neuropsychology ★

Division 40 of the American Psychological Association is a scientific and professional forum for psychologists interested in the study of brain-behavior relationships.

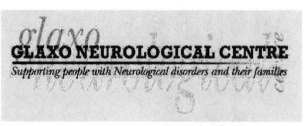

- Action for Dysphasic Adults
- Alzheimers Disease Society
- ANTS(syringomyelia)
- Arachnoiditis Trust
- Assoc. Of Spina Bifida and Hydrocephalus
- Ataxia Support Group
- British Brain Tumour Assoc.
- Charcot Marie Tooth
- Different Strokes
- Dystonia Society
- Encephalitis Support
- Guillain Barre Synd. Support Group
- Headway(head injuries)
- Huntington's Disease Assoc.
- Jennifer Trust for Spinal Muscular Atrophy
- Meningitis Merseyside

- Mersey Region Epilepsy Assoc.
- Motor Neurone Disease Association.
- Multiple Sclerosis Research Trust
- Multiple Sclerosis Society
- Muscular Dystrophy Society
- M.E. Assoc.
- Myasthenia Gravis Assoc.
- National Meningitis Trust
- Neurofibromatosis Assoc.
- Parkinson Disease Society
- Pick's Disease Support Group
- P.S.P.Europe(progressive supranuclear palsy)
- SCOPE(cerebral palsy)
- Spinal Injuries Association
- Stroke Assoc.
- Tourette's Syndrome Assoc.
- Tuberous Sclerosis Assoc.

<http://glaxocentre.merseyside.org/>
Glaxo Neurological Centre
Liverpool, England

A unique non-medical advice and information center for people with neurological conditions and those who care for them.

<http://cns-web.bu.edu/inns/>
International Neural Network Society
Woodbury, New Jersey

Seeking to learn about and advance our understanding of the modeling of behavioral and brain processes and the application of neural modeling concepts to technological problems.

<http://www.med.ohio-state.edu/ins/index.html>
The International Neuropsychological Society
Columbus, Ohio

Promoting research, education, and service in neuropsychology with more than 3,500 members throughout the world.

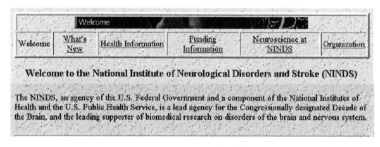

Welcome to the National Institute of Neurological Disorders and Stroke (NINDS)

The NINDS, an agency of the U.S. Federal Government and a component of the National Institutes of Health and the U.S. Public Health Service, is a lead agency for the Congressionally designated Decade of the Brain, and the leading supporter of biomedical research on disorders of the brain and nervous system.

<http://www.ninds.nih.gov/welcomhp.htm>
National Institute of Neurological Disorders and Stroke (NINDS) ★★
National Institutes of Health, Bethesda, Maryland

- NINDS:
  Coordinates research on the causes, prevention, diagnosis, and treatment of neurological disorders and stroke
  Provides grants-in-aid to public and private institutions and to individuals

Operates a program for the funding of research in certain areas of need
Provides individual and institutional fellowships
Conducts intramural and collaborative research
Collects and disseminates research information

- A keyword search engine allows for the retrieval of articles, organizations, and other information.

<http://www.premier.net /~cogito/neuropsy.html>
Neuropsychology Central ★★
Cyber Rehab Services of Baton Rouge, Louisiana

- This site's objectives are: to increase public knowledge of neuropsychology as a branch of practical medicine; to indicate the contribution which neuropsychology is making to the neurosciences; to describe the importance of neuropsychology as a science of brain and behavior; to act as a resource for the professional and layperson alike.
- The links, many of which are reviewed, are organized by category including Assessment, Developmental, Treatment, Geriatric, Software, Home Pages, Cognitive, Newsgroups, Navigation, Neuroscience, On-line Forums, Organizations, Neuroimaging, Forensics, Medical, Training, Mailgroups, Laboratories, Publications, Psychology.
- This site has a general psychology search engine listed in Chapter 2.

<http://www.flash.net/~jhom/Links.htm>
Neuropsychology Links ★
Links to many related NP web sites, from the Neuropsychology Center

<http://www.neuroguide.com>
Neurosciences on the Internet ★★
Sponsored by RBI Neurochemicals and the *Neuroscientist Journal*

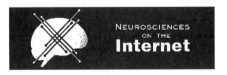

- Resources can be searched by keyword.
- Sections include:

Neurobiology	Psychiatry
Neurology	Psychology
Neurosurgery	Cognitive Sciences

<http://www.bic.mni.mcgill.ca/>
McConnell Brain Imaging Centre
Montreal Neurological Institute, McGill University

- BIC is one of the largest scientific communities in North
- America dedicated solely to research imaging of the human brain.
- The program emphasizes quantitative 3-D investigation of brain structure and function.

<http://www.nan.drexel.edu/>
The National Academy of Neuropsychology
Aurora, Colorado
- More than 3,000 members, mostly clinical neuropsychologists.
- Dedicated to the advancement of knowledge in the understanding, assessment, and remediation of brain dysfunction.

B. *Computers and Mental Health*

 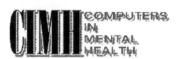 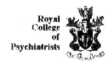

<http://www.ex.ac.uk/cimh/welcome.htm>
Computers in Mental Health ★★
The Royal College of Psychiatrists, University of Exeter, UK
- The site includes:
  Software Information and Reviews
  Software Suppliers, Mental Health Software
  Sites, Books and Journals
  Articles and Papers
  Archives
  Other Resources
- An alphabetical listing of software titles is available using the software A-Z option.

<http://plaid.hawk.plattsburgh.edu/psychlink>
PsycLink ★★
Peter Hornby and Psychology Department, State University of New York at Plattsburgh
   The site includes comprehensive information about psychology software and WWW resources including:
     A Catalog of descriptive information about psychology software
     Directory of software users
     Archive for PC software
     Announcement service available to users

<http://www.york.ac.uk/inst/ctipsych/web/MainMenu.html>
CTI Centre for Psychology ★★
University of York, UK
> This site contains information on:
>> Publications including *Psychology Software News*
>> On-line resources for teaching and learning psychology
>> Software distribution service and a directory of psychology software
>> Workshops and conferences
>> Info on all 24 CTI Centres
>> Set of links to resources for teaching statistics
>> Selection of on-line resources categorized by psychology topic

<http://www.ppig.org.>
The Psychology of Programming Interest Group
Judith Segal, University of Surrey, Guildford, England
> Established in 1987 to bring together people from diverse communities to explore common interests in the psychological aspects of programming and/or in the computational aspects of psychology.

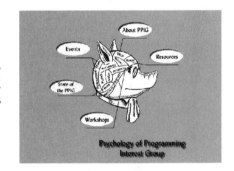

<http://www.lafayette.edu/allanr/scip.html>
The Society for Computers in Psychology
A non-profit organization of researchers interested in applications of computers in psychology.

C. *Associations, Organizations, and Institutes*

The headquarters of some of these organizations may shift from time to time as new officers are appointed.

i. PSYCHOLOGY-RELATED

<http://www.electriciti.com/aafp/>
American Academy of Forensic Psychology
Pittsburgh, Pennsylvania
> The American Board of Professional Psychology awards the Diplomate in Forensic Psychology through the AAFP to licensed Ph.D. psychologists in the United States and Canada.

Forensic Psychology is the application of the science and profession of psychology to questions and issues relating to law and the legal system. The word "forensic" comes from the Latin word "forensis," meaning "of the forum," where the law courts of ancient Rome were held. Today forensic refers to the application of scientific principles and practices to the adversary process where specially knowledgeable scientists play a role.

<http://www.aamft.org>
American Association for Marriage and Family Therapy
Washington, D.C.
> • Established in 1942, the AAMFT works to advance the marriage and family therapy profession as a means of promoting marital and family well-being.
> • The AAMFT establishes guidelines and standards for education, supervision, ethics, and clinical practice.

American Association for Marriage and Family Therapy
Building the Future for Marriage and Family Therapy

AMERICAN ASSOCIATION *of* PASTORAL COUNSELORS

> A recent Gallup poll found that when confronted with a personal problem needing counseling or psychotherapy, 66% of persons would prefer a therapist who represented spiritual values and beliefs, and 81% would prefer a therapist who enabled them to integrate their values and belief system into the counseling process.

<http://www.metanoia.org/aapc/>
American Association of Pastoral Counselors
Fairfax, Virginia
- Founded in 1963
- A recent Gallup Poll found that when confronted with a personal problem needing counseling, 66 percent of persons would prefer a therapist who represented spiritual values, and 81 percent would prefer a therapist who enabled them to integrate their values and belief system into the counseling process.
- Pastoral counselors have received specialized graduate training in both religion and the behavioral sciences.

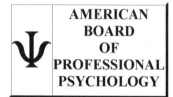

AMERICAN BOARD OF PROFESSIONAL PSYCHOLOGY

<http://www.biof.com/americanpsychology.html>
American Board of Professional Psychology
Colombia, Missouri
ABPP offers certification as a specialist in the areas of behavioral psychology, clinical psychology, clinical neuropsychology, counseling psychology, family psychology, forensic psychology, health psychology, industrial/organizational psychology, school psychology.

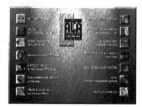

<http://www.counseling.org/>
The American Counseling Association
Alexandria, Virginia
- Leadership training, continuing education, and advocacy services to 55,000 members.
- ACA has World Counseling Chat for members and visitors.

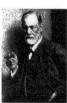

<http://apsa.org/>
The American Psychoanalytic Association ★★
New York, New York
- The APA has a searchable index of more than 30,000 entries from psychoanalytic journal articles, books, and book reviews. The index can be searched by keywords, and reprints can be ordered by phone, fax, or e-mail.
- The APA is a Regional Association of the International Psychoanalytic Association.

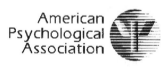

American Psychological Association

<http://www.apa.org>
American Psychological Association ★★
Washington, D.C.
The search engine features of the APA are referenced in the Psychology/Psychiatry Chapter 2.

<http://psych.hanover.edu/APS/>
American Psychological Society
Washington, D.C.

> With nearly 15,000 members, the APA is the most active and rapidly growing scientific society in the world dedicated to advancing the best of scientific psychology in research, application, and the improvement of the human condition.

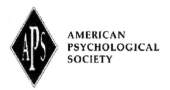

AMERICAN
PSYCHOLOGICAL
SOCIETY

<http://www.abpsi.org/>
The Association of Black Psychologists
Washington, D.C.

> The ABP sees its mission and destiny as the liberation of the African Mind, empowerment of the African Character, and enlivement and illumination of the African Spirit. It currently has over 1,400 members.

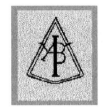

<http://www.aatbs.com/>
Association for Advanced Training in the Behavioral Sciences

> The AATBS is the oldest provider of review programs for licensure exams in the mental health fields. More than 50,000 mental health professionals have attended their workshops and used their studying materials.

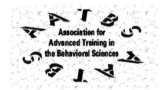

<http://www.psy.uva.nl/ResEdu/KP/Div/ALGP1.shtml>
Associations of Lesbian and Gay Psychologists in Europe
Trier, Germany

> Works to combat homophobia, support gay and lesbian affirmative action, and advance the health of lesbians and gay men.

Associations of Lesbian and Gay Psychologists in Europe

<http://www.iop.bpmf.ac.uk/home/trust/ot/aotmh.htm>
Association of Occupational Therapists
London, England

> The AOTMH works to bring together ideas and experience of OT's working in all fields of mental health. It focuses on alcohol and substance misuse, community mental health, forensic psychiatry, general mental health, homelessness.

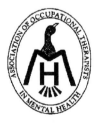

<http://www.bhs.mq.edu.au/aps/>
The Australian Psychological Society ★
Carlton, VIC

> APS has over 11,600 members. There is also a mini psychology search engine and information on:
> Careers in psychology
> Institutions, organizations, and publications
> Patient care: a guide for medical practitioners
> Psychological perspectives on euthanasia and the terminally ill

The Australian Psychological Society

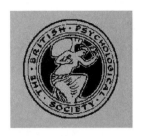

<http://www.bps.org.uk/>
The British Psychological Society
London, England
- Founded in 1901, the Society has 27,000 members.
- Branches are located in North of England, Northern Ireland, Scotland, Wales, Wessex and Wight, and the West Midlands. Regional offices are located in Scotland, Northern Ireland, and Wales.

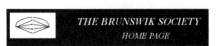

<http://www.albany.edu/cpr/brunswik/>
The Brunswik Society
The State University of New York at Albany
An informal association of researchers interested in understanding and improving human judgment and decision making.

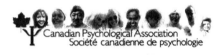

<http://www.cpa.ca/>
The Canadian Psychological Association ★
Ottawa, Ontario, Canada
- The CPA site has a psychology search engine.
- Text is available in English or French.
- Table of contents and abstracts are listed for CPA's three journals.

EFPPA
European Federation of Profesional Psychologists Association
Fédération Européenne des Associations de Psychologues
Europäische Föderation des Berusfsverbände von Psychologen

<http://www.cop.es/efppa/english/>
European Federation of Professional Psychologists Association
Officers and task forces are located throughout Europe.
Founded in 1981, there are 26 member associations representing 100,000 psychologists.

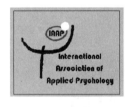

<http://www.ucm.es/OTROS/Psyap/iaap/>
International Association of Applied Psychology
Universidad Complutense, Madrid
- IAAP sponsors the International Congress of Applied Psychology every four years.
- The IAAP award is given to colleagues who have made important contributions.

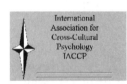

<http://www.fit.edu/CampusLife/clubs-org/iaccp/>
International Association for Cross-Cultural Psychology
Florida Institute of Technology, Melbourne, Florida
IACCP was founded in 1972 and has a membership of over 500 persons in more than 65 countries.

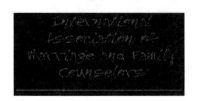

<http://familycounselors.org/>
International Association of Marriage and Family Counselors ★
Alexandria, Virginia
- A division of the American Counseling Association.
- Offers a series of videotapes demonstrating couple counseling.
- Links to related resources.

<http://www.bioenergetic-therapy.com/>
The International Institute for Bioenergetic Analysis
New York, New York
    Dedicated to the practice of mind/body psychotherapy.

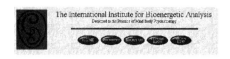

<http://134.173.117.152/>
International Society of Political Psychology ★
Minneapolis, Minnesota
- ISPP seeks to facilitate communication across disciplinary, geographic and political boundaries among scholars, concerned individuals in government and public posts, the communications media, and elsewhere who have a scientific interest in the relationship between politics and psychological processes.
- A search engine lists WWW resources for political psychologists.

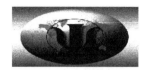

ISPP HOMEPAGE
Welcome to the International Society of Political Psychology's Homepage

<http://www.mentalhealth.org.uk/>
The Mental Health Foundation ★
United Kingdom
- A charity dedicated to improving the lives of people with mental health problems or learning disabilities.
- Information on programs, publications, and conferences.

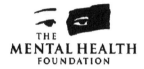

<http://www.naspweb.org/>
National Association of School Psychologists ★
Bethesda, Maryland
    Includes links to useful school psychology sites.

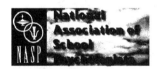

National Mental Health Association

<http://www.nmha.org/>
National Mental Health Association
Alexandria, Virginia
- Founded in 1909, NMHA has more than 300 affiliates throughout America.
- The NMHA is the only citizen-volunteer advocacy organization dedicated to addressing mental health issues.

Working for America's Mental Health

<http://www.uis.edu/~radpsy/>
Radical Psychology Network
Dennis Fox, University of Illinois at Springfield
- Radical psychologists want to work politically to improve social conditions.
- RPN believes enhancing human welfare demands fundamental social change.

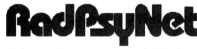

Notices   Documents   Books & Reviews
Administration   Links   Archives   Home

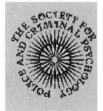

<http://www.wesleyan.edu/spn>
Social Psychology Network ★★
Scott Plous, Wesleyan University, Middletown, Connecticut
- SPN is a comprehensive resource for social psychology info on the WWW.
- Web sites are listed that relate to specific social psychology topics.
- Social psychology doctoral programs, research groups, and journals are listed.
- Home pages of individual social psychologists are listed.
- Participate in on-line social psychology studies from around the world.
- Browse through a list of textbooks and courses related to social psychology.

<http://www.jmu.edu/psyc/spcp/>
The Society for Police and Criminal Psychology
Hauppauge, New York
Encourages the application of behavioral science knowledge to problems in criminal justice.

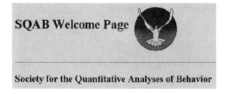

<http://www.umich.edu/~sociss>
The Society for the Psychological Study of Social Issues
Ann Arbor, Michigan
Established in 1936 with approximately 3,500 psychologists and allied scientists who share a common concern with research on the psychological aspects of important social issues.

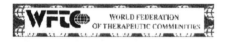

<http://www.jsu.edu/psychology/sqab.html>
Society for the Quantitative Analyses of Behavior
Jacksonville State University, Jacksonville, Alabama
Founded in 1978 to present symposia and publish material which bring a quantitative analysis to bear on the understanding of behavior.

<http://www.echonyc.com/~wftc/>
World Federation of Therapeutic Communities
New York, New York
- The WFTC seeks to join together in a worldwide association of sharing, understanding and cooperation within the global therapeutic community.
- The WFTC takes a holistic approach to the healing of human beings and encourages indigenous leadership to adapt the TC to respective cultures.

ii. PSYCHIATRY AND MEDICINE-RELATED

<http://www.mcn.com/aoop.htm>
Academy of Organizational and Occupational Psychiatry
McLean, Virginia
> Founded in 1990, the AOOP was created to provide a forum for exchanging ideas between psychiatry and the world of work.

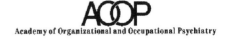

<http://www.apm.org/>
The Academy of Psychosomatic Medicine
Chicago, Illinois
> Established in 1954 to focus on patients with comorbid medical and psychiatric illness and the interaction between them.

<http://www.teleport.com/~amrta/>
Health WWWeb: The Alchemical Medicine Research and Teaching Association ★
Beaverton, Oregon
> - To embrace and weave together the intuitive and the technical, ancient traditions and modern science.
> - AMRTA is dedicated to altering the predominant 'symptom-oriented' approach to health care by promoting natural medicine and alternative therapies which address the deeper causes of illness, and which treat the body, spirit, and mind as an integrated whole.

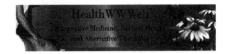

<http://www.aacap.org/web/aacap/>
American Academy of Child and Adolescent Psychiatry ★
Washington, D.C.
> - The AACAP provides this important information as a public service to assist parents and families in their most important roles. They add that it is neither ethical nor responsible to use the Internet for consultation about specific children or families.
> - *Facts for Families* has 56 fact sheets in English and Spanish on a variety of issues; they may be duplicated and distributed free of charge as long as the AACAP is properly credited and no profit is gained from their use.

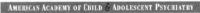
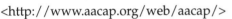

<http://www.aagpgpa.org/home.html>
The American Association for Geriatric Psychiatry
Bethesda, Maryland
> The AAGP represents over 1,500 geriatric psychiatrists in the United States and abroad.

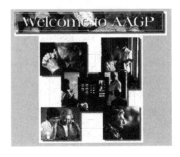

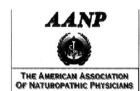

<http://www.infinite.org/Naturopathic.Physician/Welcome.html>

The American Association of Naturopathic Physicians ★

Seattle, Washington

  Sections on with links to:
    Finding a N.D.
    N.D. Education
    Politics
    General Information

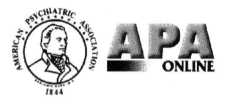

<http://www.ama-assn.org/>

The American Medical Association ★★

Chicago, Illinois

  • Health Insight has information for consumers.
  • Links are available to other Internet medical sites.
  • Public areas of the site may be searched by keyword.
  • A variety of abstracts and full-text articles can be searched by keyword in the Search feature.

<http://www.psych.org/main.html>

The American Psychiatric Association ★★

Washington, D.C.

  The APA site provides information for psychiatrists, mental-health providers, and patients on virtually all aspects of mental illness and the therapeutic process. Some of the site's categories include:
    Public Policy Advocacy
    News and Media
    Clinical Resources
    Research Resources
    Public Information
    APA Members
    Other Organizations
    Medical Education
    Practice of Psychiatry
    Library and Publications

The American Psychiatric Association is a national medical specialty society whose 40,500 physician members specialize in the diagnosis and treatment of mental and emotional illnesses and substance use disorders.

The American Psychiatric Nurses Association

<http://www.apna.org/>

The American Psychiatric Nurses Association ★

Washington, D.C.

  Information about APNA and links to other web sites.

The International Association for Near – Death Studies

<http://www.iands.org>

International Association for Near-Death Studies ★

East Windsor Hill, Connecticut

  Information for anyone with an interest in near-death experiences.

<http://rdz.stjohns.edu/iasp/>
International Association of Spiritual Psychiatry
Haifa, Israel

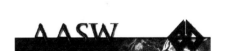

- IASP, founded in 1994, works to create a psycho-spiritual medicine integrating scientific thought and mystical insight.
- Information is available in English and French.
- Membership is open to non-health professionals.

<http://web.pnhp.org/pnhp/index.html>
Physicians for a National Health Program
Chicago, Illinois

- PNHP is a single issue organization advocating a universal, comprehensive single-payer national health care program.
- PNHP members have diverse political orientations.

<http://socbehmed.org/sbm/sbm.htm>
Society of Behavioral Medicine
Rockville, Maryland

SBM has created the premier scientific forum for over 3,000 behavioral and biomedical researchers and clinicians to study the interactions of behavior, physiological and biochemical states, and morbidity and mortality.

iii. SOCIAL WORK

<http://www.aasw.asn.au/>
Australian Association of Social Workers ★

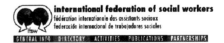

Kingston, Australian Capital Territory with branches located throughout Australia and New South Wales

Links to social work sources worldwide are organized alphabetically.

<http://www.cswf.org/>
Clinical Social Work Federation Inc. (formerly the National Federation of Societies for Clinical Social Work)
CSWF has 31 state societies in the United States

<http://www.ifsw.org/>
International Federation of Social Workers
Oslo, Norway

Represented in 59 countries with more than 435,000 social workers.

<http://homepages.iol.ie/~iasw/>
Irish Association of Social Workers
Dublin, Ireland

Founded in 1971 with eight regional branches throughout Ireland.

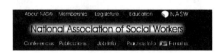

<http://www.naswdc.org/>
The National Association of Social Workers
Washington, D.C.
> Founded in 1955 with over 155,000 members throughout the United States, Puerto Rico, the Virgin Island, and abroad.

<http://www.nisw.org.uk/>
National Institute for Social Work
London, England
> To identify and promote good practice and management in social work and social care.

D. *Treatment Orientations and Modalities*

Web sites listed below represent traditional and nontraditional forms of therapy. Their listing does not necessarily constitute an endorsement of their practices or methods.

i. ACUPRESSURE AND ACUPUNCTURE

<http://www.acupuncture.com/>
Acupuncture.com ★
Yo San University, Santa Monica, California
> Categories include:
> Consumer resources
> Practitioner resources
> Student resources
> Marketplace

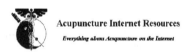

<http://www.med.auth.gr/%7Ekaranik/english/links.htm
Acupuncture Internet Resources ★★
> Everything about Acupuncture on the World Wide Web

<http://www.hightouchnet.com/p2.html>
High Touch: A Gentle Form of Acupressure
> Books, instructional teaching aids, and information on certification.

ii. ALEXANDER TECHNIQUE

<http://www.life.uinc.edu/jeff/alextech.html>
The Alexander Technique ★
> Internet resources and mailing lists.

<http://www.pavilion.co.uk/stat/>
The Society of Teachers of the Alexander Technique
London, England
- The Alexander Technique, developed by F.M. Alexander, is a system of postural reintegration which can relieve pain and stress by restoring to our bodies a balanced, regenerative, natural poise.
- Mail order books and a list of accredited teachers are available.

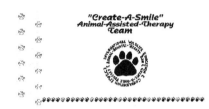

Established 1958

The Society of Teachers of the Alexander Technique

20 London House, 266 Fulham Road, London, SW10 9EL

iii. ANIMAL-ASSISTED THERAPY

<http://www.aat.org/>
"Create-A-Smile" Animal-Assisted-Therapy Team
Los Angeles, California
- Promoting the animal-human bond and its healing benefit.
- Creating Animal-Assisted-Therapy teams around the world.

<http://www.instanet.com/~sert/mainpage.html>
Special Equestrian-Riding Therapy Inc.
Malibu Creek State Park, California
SERT was founded in 1987 by a group of parents with disabled children.

iv. ART THERAPY

<http://www.sofer.com/art-therapy/>
Art Therapy on the Web ★
Art therapy links, articles, and vacancies.

Art Therapy on the Web

Home Page
Introduction   *W*elcome to Art Therapy on
Art Therapy Links   the Web.
Art Therapy Articles   Last Updated: February 18th, 1997
Art Therapy Vacancies   Art Therapy Noticeboard
Art Therapy Noticeboard   This site is a free resource for the art therapy community.

v. BIBLICAL THERAPY

<http://www.ibtonline.org>
Institute of Biblical Therapy
Huntsville, Alabama
Provide treatment, at or above professional standards, structured on biblical truths combined with solid therapeutic techniques that strengthen your relationship with Jesus Christ.

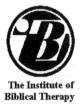

The Institute of Biblical Therapy

vi. BIOFEEDBACK

<http://www.aapb.org/index.htm>
Association for Applied Psychophysiology and Biofeedback ★
Wheat Ridge, Colorado
Advance the development, dissemination and utilization of knowledge about applied psychophysiology and biofeedback to improve the health and quality of life through research, education and practice.

<http://www.bfe.org/>
Biofeedback Foundation of Europe
Woerden, the Netherlands
>   Promote a greater awareness of biofeedback among European health professionals.

<http://www.webideas.com/biofeedback/about.htm>
Biofeedback Webzine
>   An online magazine dedicated to providing information and forums about biofeedback.

<http://freud.tau.ac.il/~biosee/>
The Home Page for Clinical Psychophysiologists and Biofeedback Therapists ★
>   Includes information on conferences, biofeedback equipment, diagnoses for which biofeedback is an established treatment, and related links.

vii. COGNITIVE-BEHAVIORAL THERAPY

<http://mindstreet.com/cbt.html>
Basics of Cognitive Therapy
>   Excerpted from *Cognitive Therapy: A Multimedia Learning Program.*

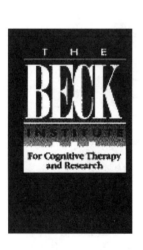

<http://www.beckinstitute.org/>
The Beck Institute for Cognitive Therapy and Research
Bala Cynwyd, Pennsylvania
>   The institute has cognitive therapy training programs for health professionals.

<http://www.cb1.com/cb1/John/public/Religion/CCT.html>
Christian Cognitive Therapy
>   Combining cognitive therapy with the Book of Proverbs.

<http://www.nacbt.org/>
National Association of Cognitive-Behavioral Therapists ★
Weirton, West Virginia
>   Links are available to general psychology sites as well as other cognitive-related URL's.

viii. COLOR THERAPY

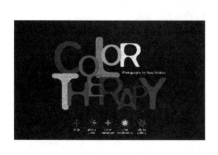

<http://myth.com/color/opening.html>
Color Therapy
>   Color meanings and meditations.

ix. DANCE THERAPY

<http://www.ADTA.org/>
American Dance Therapy Association

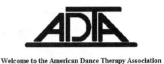

Welcome to the American Dance Therapy Association

- ADTA, founded in 1966, works to establish and maintain high standards of professional education and competence in the field of dance/movement therapy.
- There are currently five master's level training programs approved by the ADTA.

x. DRAMA THERAPY

<http://csep.sunyit.edu:80/~joel/nadt.html>
Drama Therapy

Joel Plotkin's page with information on associations, school programs, and links.

xi. EYE MOVEMENT DESENSITIZATION AND REPROCESSING (EMDR)

<http://www.emdr.com>
EMDR Institute Inc.
Pacific Grove, California

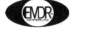

EYE MOVEMENT DESENSITIZATION AND REPROCESSING

- EMDR is an interactional, standardized approach and method that integrates into, and augments, a treatment plan. EMDR accelerates the treatment of a wide range of pathologies and self-esteem issues related to both upsetting past events and present life conditions.
- There are more controlled studies to date on EMDR than on any other method used in the treatment of trauma.
- A schedule of training sessions for certification is included.

xii. EXPRESSIVE THERAPIES

<http://www.expressivetherapy.org/etclower.html>
Expressive Therapy Concepts ★★
Mont Clare, Pennsylvania

An organization dedicated to education and service in the creative arts therapies and related disciplines (art, dance, music, poetry, drama, psychodrama).

xiii. FENG SHUI

<http://sunflower.signet.com.sg/~cecil/>
Feng Shui Made Easy
Cecil Lee, Singapore

A place to start for basic information.

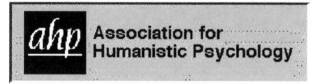

<http://www.netcomuk.co.uk/~kayers/
fengshui.html>
Feng Shui Society ★
United Kingdom
> Established in 1993 to advance Feng Shui prin-
> ciples and concepts as a contribution to the
> creation of harmonious environments for indi-
> viduals and society in general.

xiv. GESTALT THERAPY

<http://www.gestalt.org/index.htm>
The Gestalt Therapy Page ★
- From the *Gestalt Journal* and the International Gestalt Ther-
  apy Association
- Links to articles and web sites dealing with Gestalt therapy.

xv. GROUP PSYCHOTHERAPY

<http://freud.tau.ac.il/~haimw/group2.html>
Group Psychotherapy ★
> Information and links to resources for the professional group
> therapist.

xvi. HUMANISTIC PSYCHOLOGY

<http://ahpweb.bestware.net/>
The Association for Humanistic Psychology
San Francisco, California
> - An international community of people with
>   diverse talents and interests who are dedi-
>   cated to the exploration and healing of the
>   human mind, body, and soul and to build-
>   ing a society that advances our ability to
>   choose, grow, and create.
> - Membership is open to all.

xvii. HYPNOSIS

<http://www.ASCH.net/frameenh.html>
The American Society of Clinical Hypnosis
Des Plaines, Illinois
> Professional people in medicine, dentistry, psychology, social
> work, nursing, and mental health who share scientific and clin-
> ical interests in hypnosis.

<http://www.hypnosis.com/>
Hypnosis.com ★★
   Information on and links to hypnosis and Neuro-Linguistic
   Programming sites.

<http://www.infinityinst.com/>
Infinity Institute International Inc. ★
Royal Oak, Michigan
   Training, self-help hypnosis tapes, hypnosis marketing tools,
   links.

<http://www.lcch.co.uk/>
London College of Clinical Hypnosis
   Founded in 1984, LCCH teaches the application of hypnosis for
   a wide range of medical, psychological, and somatic problems.

 London College of **Clinical Hypnosis**

xviii. JUNGIAN PSYCHOLOGY

<http://www.cgjung.com/>
C. G. Jung, Analytical Psychology, and Culture
   • Home page of the *Round Table Review*
   • For those who find in Jungian psychology a profound under-
     standing of the human psyche.

<http://jungindex.net/>
The C.G. Jung Index ★★
   The site includes:
      Who's Who in Analytical Psychology
      Jungian Links on the Internet
      A C.G. Jung Picture Archive
      Essays and Papers by Jung
      Dissertations and Journal Search
      A Jungian Glossary of Terms
      An Introduction to C.G. Jung

xix. KINESIOLOGY

<http://www.lexicon.net.au/~lightman/>
Light Touch Kinesiology Home Page
Melbourne, Victoria, Australia
   • An information package describing the benefits of kinesiol-
     ogy.
   • Course information and dates.

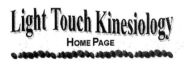

xx. MARRIAGE AND FAMILY THERAPY

<http://www.echo-on.net/~skillin/>
Marriage and Family Therapy ★
   General information for consumers and professionals.

xxi. MUSIC THERAPY

<http://members.aol.com/kathysl/index.html>
Music Therapy Info Link ★
> The site contains:
>> Schools with MT programs
>> Education and Training
>> Music Therapy links
>> FAQ's
>> Message Board

xxii. NARRATIVE THERAPY

<http://maple.lemoyne.edu/~hevern/narpsych.html>
Narrative Psychology: An Internet Guide ★
> Internet links and a guide to other narrative-based resources.

<http://www.sover.net/~mlax/>
Narrative Therapy Training
> A series of workshops conducted across North America.

xxiii. NEURO-LINGUISTIC PROGRAMMING

<http://home.earthlink.net/~jbodnar/nlpm.html>
Jeff's Favorite NLP/Hypnosis Links ★
> Links to organizations, seminars, writings on NLP.

<http://www.nlpcomprehensive.com/>
NLP Comprehensive Home Page ★
> NLP is the science of how the brain codes learning and experience. The site contains:
>> Links
>> Products
>> Training
>> Information

The Society of Neuro-Linguistic Programming™

<http://www.purenlp.com/society.htm>
The Society of Neuro-Linguistic Programming ™
San Francisco, California
> • Established in 1978 for the purpose of exerting quality control over those training programs and services claiming to represent the NLP model.
> • Information on training certification and trainers.

xxiv. ORGONOMY

<http://www.sconnect.net/~goodman/orgone.html>
Wilhelm Reich Homepage ★
- Information on Reich's life and work and Reichian therapy.
- Excerpts from the *Orgone Accumulator Handbook* by James DeMeo.

xxv. PERSONALITY

<http://www.uwinnipeg.ca/~isspr/>
International Society for the Study of Personal Relationships
University of Winnipeg, Canada

 International Society for the Study of Personal Relationships

> Formed in 1984 with the aim of stimulating and supporting scholarship and research on personal relationships, improving communication between researchers around the world engaged in the scientific study of personal relationships, and establishing the field of personal relationships within the scholarly community.

<http://fas.psych.nwu.edu/personality.html>
The Personality Project ★
Department of Psychology, Northwestern University
> The site contains:
> Links to personality research literature
> Scholarly societies
> Graduate training programs in personality
> Course syllabi from personality theory and research courses
> Special advice for students

xxvi. POLARITY THERAPY

<http://www.eclipse.co.uk/masterworks/polarity.htm>
> Individual and group training in Scotland and Norway.

Polarity Therapy Page
> Information about Randolph Stone's system of healing.

<http://www.livelinks.com/sumeria/health/polarity.html>
Polarity Therapy from the American Polarity Therapy Association
Boulder, Colorado

Energy is the vital force in the body - *Dr. Randolph Stone*
Polarity Therapy
from **The American Polarity Therapy Association**

> An introduction to PT. Body, emotions, mind and spirit are interdependent; each person shares in the responsibility for his or her own health; simple steps can be taken to improve wellness.

<http://www.eclipse.co.uk/masterworks/polarity.htm>
The Polarity Therapy Web Pages ★
> Info on P.T. and assorted links.

xxvii. PRIMAL PSYCHOTHERAPY

<http://www.primaltherapy.com/>
Dr. Arthur Janov's Primal Center
Venice, California
- Dr. Janov emphasizes that primal therapy is NOT primal scream therapy and that primal therapy is dangerous in untrained hands.
- This site has sections on:
  Applying for Therapy
  Training
  Videos and Publications
  Research
  Case Histories

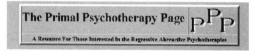

<http://www.net-connect.net/~jspeyrer/primal1.htm>
The Primal Psychotherapy Page
   Includes 54 book reviews relating to regressive psychotherapies.

xxviii. PSYCHOTHERAPY AND PSYCHOANALYSIS

<http://www.aapsa.org/>
The American Academy of Psychoanalysis
New York, New York
   AAP was founded in 1956 to provide an open forum for psychoanalysts to discuss relevant and responsible views of human behavior and to exchange ideas with psychiatric colleagues and other social and behavioral scientists.

<http://www.cyberpsych.org/apf.htm>
American Psychoanalytic Foundation
Washington, D.C.
   Dedicated to the advancement of psychoanalysis through community outreach, education, research, and clinical programs.

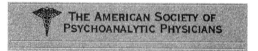

<http://pubweb.acns.nwu.edu/~chessick/aspp.htm>
The American Society of Psychoanalytic Physicians
Rockville, Maryland
- Founded in 1985 as an organization of psychoanalysts and psychoanalytically-oriented psychiatrists and physicians.
- Established to provide an open forum to further the study of psychoanalytic methods of diagnosis, treatment, and prevention of emotional disorders.

\<http://www.pccp.com.ar/apa/apa.html\>
Asociacion Psicoanalitica Argentina (The Argentina Psychoanalytic Association)
Buenos Aires, Argentina
> Founded in 1942.

\<http://www.dataweb.com.mx/apm/\>
Asociacion Psicoanalitica Mexicana (Mexican Psychoanalytic Association)
Mexico City, Mexico
> Founded in 1957.

\<http://www.psychoanalysis.asn.au/\>
Australian Psychoanalytical Society
Roseville Chase, Australia
> Founded in 1975.

\<http://www.cmps.edu\>
Center for Modern Psychoanalytic Studies
New York, New York
> Training and research in psychoanalysis since 1971.

\<http://www.mclink.it/personal/MC2038/crp2.htm#zInformation\>
Center for Research in Psychotherapy
Rome, Italy
> Information in English or Italian.

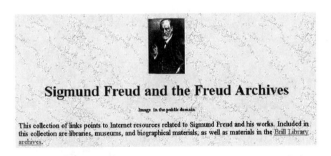

Sigmund Freud and the Freud Archives

Image in the public domain

This collection of links points to Internet resources related to Sigmund Freud and his works. Included in this collection are libraries, museums, and biographical materials, as well as materials in the Brill Library archives.

\<http://plaza.interport.net/nypsan/freudarc.html\>
Sigmund Freud and the Freud Archives ★
> A collection of Freud-related links.

\<http://www.npap.org/\>
National Psychological Association for Psychoanalysis
New York, New York
> The NPAP Training Institute was founded in 1948 and is dedicated to advancements in the practice of nonmedical psychoanalysis.

<http://www.psychoanalysis.net>
The Psychoanalytic Connection ★
> The site has sections on:
> > A Resource List for child psychotherapists
> > Listings of clinical training programs
> > Psa-Netcast is an on-line forum for psychotherapists
> > The PC helps organizations develop distance learning classes and projects
> > Links to other psychoanalytic-related sites

<http://www.sicap.it/~merciai/spi.htm>
Societa Psicoanalitica Italiana (Italian Psychoanalytic Society)
Milan, Italy
> - In Italian and English.
> - SPI maintains a national training institute.

<http://www.gallaudet.edu/~11mgourn/>
Theoretical Approaches in Psychotherapy
> Overview of various psychotherapeutic modalities and orientations.

xxix. RATIONAL-EMOTIVE BEHAVIOR THERAPY

<http://www.IRET.org/>
The Albert Ellis Institute
New York, New York
> - Founded in 1968.
> - REBT is a humanistic, action-oriented approach to emotional growth.

xxx. REIKI

<http://www.crl.com/~davidh/reiki/>
The Reiki Page ★
> Reiki (pronounced Ray-Key) is a method of natural healing based on the application of Universal Life Force Energy.

xxxi. SCHEMA-FOCUSED THERAPY

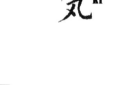

<http://www.schematherapy.com>
Schema-Focused Therapy
> Integrates cognitive therapy, behavior therapy, experiential techniques, and object relations approaches to the treatment of personality disorders, depression, and other chronic psychological problems.

xxxii. SPIRITUAL HEALING

<http://www.zip.com.au/~cee_gee/spirit.html>
Spiritual Healing/Counseling ★
Links to personal support and guidance.
> A concise summary and explanation of the world's spiritual traditions.

xxxiii. SUFI

<http://world.std.com/~habib/sufi.html>
Links to Sufi-related Resources on the Internet ★
> Sufis are mystics on the path to God; most Sufis are Muslims.

<http://sufi-psychology.org/>
The Sufi Psychology Association
Sacramento, California
> Founded by a group of psychologists, psychotherapists, psychiatrists, and researchers in related disciplines who have experience with the effects of Sufism on the human psyche.

xxxiv. THOUGHT FIELD THERAPY

<http://www.tftrx.com/>
Thought Field Therapy™
The Callahan Techniques Ltd., Indian Wells, California
> TFT is a revolutionary new method for the rapid treatment of psychological problems.

the thought field

xxxv. TRANSACTIONAL ANALYSIS

<http://www.itaa-net.org/>
The International Transactional Analysis Association
San Francisco, California
> • Facilitates international communication among people and groups who use transactional analysis.
> • Over 4,000 members in 65 countries.

ITAA
International
Transactional
Analysis
Association

xxxvi. VIDEO THERAPY

<http://www.videoimprovement.com>
The Video Improvement Program
> A video-based guidance and counseling program for adolescents and adults. VIP can be done on site with only a camcorder, a counselor, and a participant.

E. *Miscellaneous General Sites*

<http://janweb.icdi.wvu.edu/kinder/>
Americans with Disabilities Act Document Center ★
- ADA Statute.
- ADAAG (Americans with Disabilities Act Accessibility Guidelines).
- Federally Reviewed Tech Sheets.
- Other Assistance Documents.
- The Job Accommodation Network is an international toll-free service that provides information about the employability of people with disabilities.

<http://www.behavior.net/>
Behavior OnLine
BOL is the gathering place for mental health professionals. Their site's sections include:
An Editorial Corner with various articles
Ongoing discussions on many psychology-related topics
Links to Organizations, Interest Groups, and Resources

A Web Site for Counselor Educators and Supervisors

<http://www.nevada.edu/~ces/>
Counselor Educators and Supervisors Web Site ★
Internet links organized by thematic categories include:
Accreditation, Licensing and Certification
Related Professional Organizations
Counselor Education Course Information
Individual Universities' Counselor Education Department Web Pages
Grant Funding Opportunities
Publishing Companies
Research and Reference Help
Counseling and Related Software
Conferences and Seminars

<http://www.idealist.org>
ideaLIST, Action Without Borders
The Contract Center Network, New York, New York
- A worldwide directory of 10,000 not-for-profit organizations.
- Interactive system allows any nonprofit or community organization to enter and update information about its services.

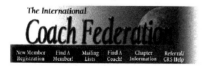

<http://www.coachfederation.org/>
The International Coach Federation
Cockeysville, Maryland
ICF has 98 chapters in 38 states and 5 countries. Personal coaching is a growing discipline that works with individual's choices, lifestyles, and career decisions.

F. *Mailing Lists*

Art Therapy Students and Professors
    Discussion List
listserv@listserv.aol.com
SUBSCRIBE ARTTHX-L

Psychological Assessment—Psychometrics
    Discussion
listserv@maelstrom.stjohns.edu
SUBSCRIBE ASSESS-L

Behavioral Health Practice
listserv@maelstrom.stjohns.edu
SUBSCRIBE PAYMED

Biofeedback and Clinical Psychology
majordomo@listp.apa.org
SUB PSYPHY Your Name

Business and Marketing for Psychotherapists
listserv@maelstrom.stjohns.edu
SUBSCRIBE PSYBUS

Collegial Chat for Psychologists at the
    PsyUSA Network
listserv@maelstrom.stjohns.edu
SUBSCRIBE PSYCHAT

Cognitive Behavior Therapy
listserv@maelstrom.stjohns.edu
SUBSCRIBE AABT-CBT

Cognitive Therapists International Associa-
    tion
listserv@listserv.kent.edu
SUBSCRIBE IACPNET

Clinical Psychologists
listserv@listserv.nodak.edu
SUBSCRIBE CLINICAL-PSYCHOLOGISTS

Community Psychology Discussion
listserv@maelstrom.stjohns.edu
SUBSCRIBE COMMPSY

Society for Computers in Psychology
listserv@psych.fullerton.edu
SUBSCRIBE SCIP-L

Credibility Assessment and Witness Psychology
listserv@idbsu.idbsu.edu
SUBSCRIBE CAAWP

Current Issues in Psychology and Psychiatry
listserv@maelstrom.stjohns.edu
SUBSCRIBE PSYCH-CI

Dialogs on Psychology
listserv@clemson.edu
SUBSCRIBE DIALOG-L

Doctor-Patient Relationship Discussions
listserv@maelstrom.stjohns.edu
SUBSCRIBE BALINT

Ecopsychology: Nature-Counseling Community
    Connection
listserv@maelstrom.stjohns.edu
SUBSCRIBE ECOPSYCHOLOGY

Education and Psychoanalysis
listserv@listserv.kent.edu
SUBSCRIBE IFPE

Educational Resources on the Internet
listserv@listserv.unb.ca
SUBSCRIBE EDRES-L

Emergency Psychiatry
listserv@maelstrom.stjohns.edu
SUBSCRIBE ERPSYCH

Enneagram
majordomo@acpub.duke.edu
SUBSCRIBE ENNEAGRAM

Exercise and Sports Psychology
listserv@vm.temple.edu
SUBSCRIBE SPORTPSY

False Memory Syndrome
http://www.mhsource.com/interactive/
    mailinglist.html
use subscription form

Forensic Psychology/Psychiatry
listserv@maelstrom.stjohns.edu
SUBSCRIBE FORENSIC-PSYCH

Grants and Contracts from NIH
listserv@list.nih.gov
SUBSCRIBE NIHGDE-L

Group Psychotherapy
majordomo@freud.apa.org
SUB GROUP-PSYCHOTHERAPY

Psych Home Care
listserv@home.ease.lsoft.com
SUBSCRIBE PSYCH-HOME-CARE

Hypnosis
listserv@maelstrom.stjohns.edu
SUBSCRIBE HYPNOSIS

Industrial Psychology
listserv@uga.cc.uga.edu
SUBSCRIBE IOOB-L

Psychology in Law Enforcement
listserv@maelstrom.stjohns.edu
SUBSCRIBE PSYCOP

Managed Behavioral Health Care
listserv@maelstrom.stjohns.edu
SUBSCRIBE MBHC

Mathematical Psychology Society
listserv@brownvm.brown.edu
SUBSCRIBE MPSYCH-L

Media and Psychology
listserv@maelstrom.stjohns.edu
SUBSCRIBE MEDIAPSY

Mental Health Workers with Bachelor's
Degree or Less (Psychiatric Technicians)
listserv@maelstrom.stjohns.edu
SUBSCRIBE MENTAL-HEALTH-WORKER

Psych News International
listserv@listserv.nodak.edu
SUBSCRIBE PSYCHNEWS

Psychiatric Nursing
listserv@maelstrom.stjohns.edu
SUBSCRIBE PSYNURSE

Psychiatric Nursing
mailbase@mailbase.ac.uk
JOIN PSYCHIATRIC-NURSING

Psychological Psychiatry
listserv@maelstrom.stjohns.edu
SUBSCRIBE PSYCHIATRY

Psychoanalysis
listserv@maelstrom.stjohns.edu
SUBSCRIBE PSYCHOAN

Psychological Services on the Internet
listserv@maelstrom.stjohns.edu
SUBSCRIBE NETPSY

Psychiatric Social Workers
listserv@maelstrom.stjohns.edu
SUBSCRIBE PSYC-SOC

Psychotherapists in Training Discussion
listserv@maelstrom.stjohns.edu
SUBSCRIBE PIT-D

APA Research Psychology Network
listserv@vtvm1.cc.vt.edu
SUBSCRIBE APASD-L

Self-Help and Psychology Magazine
listserv@maelstrom.stjohns.edu
SUBSCRIBE SHPM

Solution Focused Therapy
listserv@maelstrom.stjohns.edu
SUBSCRIBE SFT-L

American Psychological Society Student
   Caucus
listserv@vm1.mcgill.ca
SUBSCRIBE APSSCNET

Psychology and Technology
listserv@maelstrom.stjohns.edu
SUBSCRIBE PSYTECH

Transcultural Psychology
listserv@listserv.nodak.edu
SUBSCRIBE TRANSCULTURAL-PSYCHOLOGY

Chapter 4

Medical Sites of Interest

A. *Pharmacology and Psychopharmacology Search Engines*

(Use these sites to find information on specific drugs.)

RxList - The Internet Drug Index

- **KEYWORD SEARCH**
  Actions/Interactions/Brands

- **RXLIST-ID:**
  Search by Imprint Codes NEW!

- **THE TOP 200 - '96** NEW!

- **THE TOP 200 - '95**

- **KNOWN LINKS TO RXLIST**

- **ABOUT RXLIST:**
  Site Information For New Visitors

- **DAILY WWW STATS**

- **STATISTICAL SUMMARY**

- **MINI-SURVEY**

- **RXLAUGHS - WEEKLY COMIX** NEW!

\<http://www.rxlist.com>
RxList ★★
Neil Sandow, Pharm.D.
- A free service to be used only as a supplement to the advice of a physician.
- Information on hundreds of drugs including the Top 200 Prescriptions section. These 200 make up nearly two-thirds of all prescriptions filled in the United States.
- A "fuzzy" keyword search allows for incorrect spelling.
- The RxList ID feature allows unknown capsules and tablets to be identified by their ID Imprint Codes.
- Links are available to other medicine-related sites.
- RxList gets 1.5 million hits per year

MD Drugs™

The Interactive Drugs Database

<http://php2.silverplatter.com/physicians/md-drugs.htm>
MD Drugs: The Interactive Drug Database ★★
Lexi-Comp, SilverPlatter

Searchable database contains information on more than 800 prescription drugs including:
Brand Name
Therapeutic Use
Pregnancy Risk Factor
Contraindications
Warnings
Adverse Reactions
Overdosage/Toxicology
Drug Interactions
Mechanisms of Action
Usual Dosage
Reference Range
Patient Information
Nursing Implications
Dosage Forms
Stability

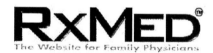

WELCOME TO RxMED. THIS IS THE COMPREHENSIVE,
PEER-REVIEWED RESOURCE FOR PRIMARY CARE PHYSICIANS,
DRUG AND ILLNESS INFORMATION AND MUCH MORE

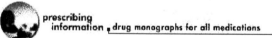

prescribing
information   drug monographs for all medications

<http://www.rxmed.com/>
RxMed: The Website for Family Physicians ★★
- From a coalition of family physicians
- Drug monographs for many medications.
- Patient handouts for over 400 illnesses.
- Employment opportunities in the medical industry.
- Information on all the shots that patients need for traveling.
- Links to health organizations and government agencies.

Clinical Pharmacology Online

<http://www.cponline.gsm.com/>
Clinical Pharmacology Online ★★
Gold Standard Multimedia, Inc.
- Full monographs describing the most common and classic medications.
- Subscription provides keyword searching, IV admixtures checking, and other features.

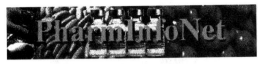

Pharmaceutical
Information
Network

<http://pharminfo.com/>
PharmInfo Net ★★
VirSci Corporation
- The PharmInfo Net DrugDB is a database of information about drugs.
- Drugs are listed alphabetically by generic names and trade-names in two separate sections.
- Each entry includes:
  Generic name
  Trade name
  Manufacturer
  Therapeutic class
  Indications
  Links to relevant articles and archives

<http://www.druginfonet.com/>
Drug Infonet: The Internet Source for Healthcare Information ★★
Drug Infonet, Inc.
- Drug Information has pharmaceutical product information and drug interactions.
- Disease Information includes individual disease descriptions.
- The Drug InfoNet archives can be searched by keyword.

- **Brand Name** - Product information listed by brand name including generic name and manufacturer.
- **Generic Name** - Product information listed by generic name including brand name and manufacturer.
- **Manufacturer** - Product information listed by pharmaceutical manufacturer.
- **Therapeutic Class** - Product information listed by therapeutic class including brand name, generic name and manufacturer.

DRUG INFONET℠

<http://www.healthtouch.com/>
Healthtouch Online ★★
Medical Strategies, Inc.
- Drug Information section has mo than 7,000 prescription drugs, ar OTC drug information comes fro Medi-Span.
- Product Information has material (products from the manufacturers.
- Drugs can be searched by keyworc

Health*touch*
Online *for better health*

Drug Information

This section enables you to find information about more than 7,000 prescription and over-the-counter medications, including common uses of a drug, the proper ways to use the medicine, possible side effects, and other helpful information. It is best to discuss this medication information with your pharmacist, doctor, or other health professional to find out how it applies to you and your particular case. The information is provided by Medi-Span®, one of the nation's most respected sources of drug and medication information.

\<http://www.healthanswers.com/health_answers/usp_drug_search/uspagif.htm\>

U.S. Pharmacopeia ★★

U.S. Pharmacopeia is a not-for-profit organization.
- Choose from easy-to-read or detailed drug information.
- USP has provided information on drugs and drug products since l820.
- Peer-reviewed evaluations.
- A keyword search is available.

\<http://home.intekom.com/pharm/\>

South African Electronic Package Inserts ★★

Malahyde Information Systems
- Makes the package inserts for South African medicines available in electronic format.
- Search by generic name, trade name, or classification.

\<http://www3.pitt.edu/~jalvin/\>

Pharmacology Home Page ★★

University of Pittsburgh Department of Pharmacology
- Drugs indexed by brand or generic name.
- Links to other pharm-related sites.

\<http://www.pharmweb.net/\>

Pharm Web ★★

Pharm Web has multiple contributors and sponsors
- A to Z listings of multiple topics related to pharmacology and pharmacy-related matters.
- A variety of discussion groups.
- Links to many other pharm-related sites.

\<http://www.medicinenet.com/\>

Medicine Net ★★

Information Network Inc.
- The Pharmacy section lists medications and side effects.
- A Medical Dictionary defines medical terms.
- Diseases and Treatments are listed in alphabetical order.
- Links are available to related sites.

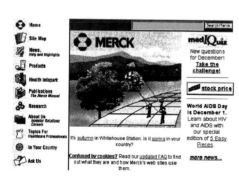

\<http://www.merck.com\>

Merck & Co. Inc. ★★

The official web site of this company includes an on-line version of the *Merck Manual*.

\<http://www.umdnj.edu/psyevnts/psychopharm.html\>

Psychopharmacology Resources ★

Dr. Myron Pulier, University of Dentistry and Medicine of New Jersey

Links to several pharmacy- and substance abuse-related web sites.

<http://www.cmhc.com:80/guide/pro22.htm#lith>
Psychopharmacology and Drug References
Mental Health Net (main site referenced in Chapter Two)
- An A to Z listing of commonly used psychiatric medications.
- Links to sites that provide drug references and databases.
- Links to drug-related journals, publications, and research papers.
- Other resources.

<http://www.geocities.com/HotSprings/2836/meds.html.>
Psychiatric Medications ★
Sarah Pleasant
    Medications listed by category.

<http://www.uct.ac.za/depts/pha/samfhtml.htm>
South African Medicines Formulary ★★ (electronic version)
Department of Pharmacology, University of Cape Town

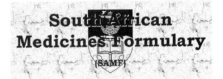

- Material may be used for educational purposes and by not-for-profit enterprises.
- A keyword search is available.
- Pharmacological agents are grouped by their relevance to:
    Alimentary tract and metabolism
    Blood and blood forming organs
    Cardiovascular system
    Dermatologicals
    Genitourinary system and sex hormones
    Systemic hormonal preparations (excluding sex hormones)
    General anti-infectives for systemic use
    Antineoplastic and immunomodulating agents
    Musculoskeletal system
    Central nervous system
    Antiparasitic products
    Respiratory system
    Sensory organs
    Various

<http://www.fda.gov/fdahomepage.html>
Food and Drug Administration ★
United States Government
    Includes information on:
        Human Drugs
        Foods
        Animal Drugs
        Toxicology
        Children and Tobacco
        Medical Devices/Radiological Health
        Biologics
        Cosmetics

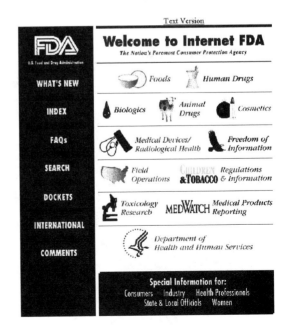

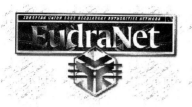

Network Services for the European Union Pharmaceutical Regulatory Sector

<http://www.eudra.org/etomep/etomep.html>
European Technical Office for Medicinal Products: EudraNet ★★
European Commission—Joint Research Centre, European Commission Directorate General for Industry, European Agency for the Evaluation of Medicinal Products, the EU National Regulatory Authorities
- EudraLEX is a document system giving on-line access to European Commission legislative material.
- EudraMAT is a database with economic information about medicinal products sold commercially in the EU.
- EudraWATCH involves data loading for national pharmacovigilance centres.
- MANSEV is a network-based system for the submission of market authorizations for medicinal products by the industrial users and evaluation by regulatory users.
- EPI is a database with snoptic information on all authorized products.
- ECPHIN is a Medicinal Products Database for the EU.

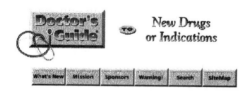

<http://pslgroup.com/NEWDRUGS.HTM>
Doctor's Guide to New Drugs or Indications ★
P/S/L Consulting Group
News found on the Internet relating to the approval of new drugs or of new indications for previously available drugs.

B. *Clinical Trials, Taking Medications, and Basic Pharmacy Information*

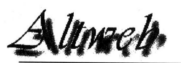

Center For Alternatives To Animal Testing

<http://www.sph.jhu.edu/~altweb/
Altweb: Center for Alternatives to Animal Testing
School of Public Health, Johns Hopkins University
- News, information, discussion, and resources from the field of alternatives to animal testing.
- Funded by the Alternatives Research and Development Foundation, the Doerenkamp-Zbinden Foundation, the Humane Society of the United States, the Office for Protection from Research Risks at the National Institutes of Health, and the Proctor and Gamble Co.

<http://www.centerwatch.com/>
Center Watch: Clinical Trials Listing Service
- An international listing of clinical research trials.
- Learn about drug therapies newly approved by the FDA.
- E-mail notification service informs subscribers of future postings in a particular therapeutic area.

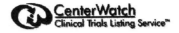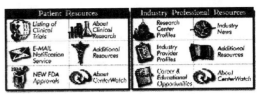

Welcome to the CenterWatch Clinical Trials Listing Service. You can use this web site to find a variety of information related to clinical trials. Our web site is designed to be a resource both for patients interested in participating in clinical trials and for research professionals. Please send us any suggestions on how we can continue to improve this service.

<http://www.healthtouch.com/level1/leaflets/103068/103068.htm>
Guide to Taking Medications ★
Medical Strategies, Inc.
> Helpful tips and charts on many aspects of taking meds.

<http://www.ns.net/users/ryan/rxabrv.html>
How to Read the Prescription
Ryan G. Seo, Pharm.D.
> The list of commonly used medical abbreviations which are normally seen on doctor's prescriptions.

<http://www.geohealthweb.com/ISMP/>
The Institute for Safe Medication Practices
Warminster, Pennsylvania
> ISMP works closely with healthcare practitioners and institutions, regulatory agencies, professional organizations and the pharmaceutical industry to provide education about adverse drug events and their prevention.

<http://www.mercator-hs.be/medisch/welcome.html>
Multilingual Glossary of Technical and Popular Medical Terms
Heymans Institute of Pharmacology, University of Gent; Mercator School, Department of Applied Linguists
> Medical terms in nine European languages

<http://med-www.bu.edu/pharmacology/Programmed/glossary.html>
Glossary of Terms and Symbols Used in Pharmacology
Boston University School of Medicine Department of Pharmacology and Experimental Therapeutics
> An A to Z index with comprehensive descriptions.

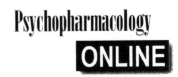

<http://www.hatherleigh.com/Psychoph.htm>
Psychopharmacology Online
Hatherleigh Company, Ltd.
> Interactive web site devoted to the advancement of the science of psychopharmacology.

Welcome to the only website devoted to the advancement of the science of psychopharmacology. Designed for clinicians and allied health professionals, in its pages you'll find the tools you need to stay abreast in this rapidly changing field. We welcome your ideas, comments, suggestions, and most of all, your interaction.

<http://www.pharmacy.co.nz/companies/index.cfm>
Pharmaceutical Companies
NetSynergy Ltd.
> An alphabetical list of worldwide companies with hyperlinks to their web sites.

<http://www.cpb.uokhsc.edu/pharmacy/company.html>
Pharmacy Page
> • The Virtual Library, University of Oklahoma Health Sciences Center
> • An alphabetical list of worldwide companies with hyperlinks to their websites.

<http://ceus.com/courses/psy805.htm>
Psychopharmacology Course Online
WebEd unLtd.
> On-line course with continuing education credits.

<http://www.fairlite.com/ocd/medres/pma.shtml>
Places You Can Contact If You Cannot Afford Medication
The OCD Page
> Listings of indigent patient programs from various pharmaceutical companies.

The Medicine Program
Can't Afford Your Prescription Medication?
Free Prescription Medicine is Available to those who Qualify.

<http://ims1.ims-1.com/~freemed/>
Free Prescription Medicine to Those Who Qualify
The Medicine Program, Poplar Bluff, Missouri
> A nationwide program to help people of all ages.

<http://iuphar.pharmacology.unimelb.edu.au/>
The International Union of Pharmacology
University of Melbourne, Australia
> A member of the International Council of Scientific Unions.

<http://www.thecompounders.com/>
Professional Compounding Centers of America Inc.
Houston, Texas
> A web site to help compounding pharmacists treat unique patient needs.

<http://www.paddocklabs.com/>
Paddock Laboratories ★
> This company's website has compounding information on:
> Vehicles
> Actives
> Techniques and procedures for extemporaneous compounding
> Stability/formulation studies

C. *Toxicology, Complications, Death and Dying*

<http://www.actis.org/>
AIDS Clinical Trials Information Service
ACTIS
Rockville, Maryland
> Provides information on clinical trials for persons with AIDS and HIV infection. ACTIS maintains an on-line database on trial protocols and one on drugs.

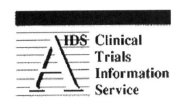

<http://www.snowcrest.net/lassen/mcsei.html>
Chemically Sensitive or Environmentally Ill Resources ★★
> Internet links to help the chemically sensitive include:
> Agencies and Advocate Groups
> Articles
> Audio
> Books
> Building Materials
> Carpet
> Catalogs
> Clothing
> Definitions
> Dental
> Doctors
> Electro Magnetics
> Food
> Homeopathy
> Laboratories
> Lawyers
> Links to pertinent sites
> Magazines
> Pest Control
> Supplements
> Video

Resources for the Chemically Sensitive or Environmentally Ill

<http://www.rights.org/deathnet/open.html>
DeathNet ★
> An international site dealing respectfully with all aspects of death and dying.

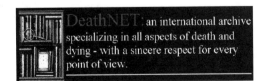

<http://www.newciv.org/worldtrans/naturaldeath.html>
The Natural Death Centre ★
London, England
> To support those dying at home and improve the quality of dying

<http://www.asf.org/index.html>
American Share Foundation ★★
Van Nuys, California

> Promoting the continuum of life through transplants and organ donations.

<http://www.vrsc.com/>
Viatical Settlement Option
VSO Corporation, Baton Rouge, Louisiana

> This program allows people with life-threatening illnesses to sell all or part of their existing life insurance policies. The amount paid is determined in part by projected life expectancy, future premiums, and current interest rates.

<http://www.ada.org/>
The American Dental Association
Chicago, Illinois

> Products, services, and consumer information, which includes ADA positions on dental amalgam.

<http://www.ephca.com/>
Chronic Illness and Chronic Mercury Exposure from Amalgams and the Environment
Environmental and Preventive Health Center of Atlanta, Georgia

> Information on mercury toxicity and other disorders.

<http://www.unpronounceable.com/amalgam/index.html>
The Crusade Against Dental Amalgam ★

> Definitions of related topics and links to resources on both sides of the controversy.

Mercury in the Mouth

<http://vest.gu.se/~bosse/Mercury/Mouth/default.html>
Mercury in the Mouth ★
Bo Walhjalt, Gothenburg, Sweden

> • Current amalgam status and restrictions around the world.
> • Resources and references with links to abstracts.

<http://www.vimy-dentistry.com/toxic.html>
Toxic Teeth: The Chronic Mercury Poisoning of Modern Man

> Information and a bibliography of dental amalgam resources.

<http://ourworld.compuserve.com/homepages/pcsol/>
UK Amalgam Page ★

> • There is now compelling evidence from reputable scientific bodies such as the WHO that, despite claims from pro-amalgam bodies such as the American and British Dental Associations, mercury is NOT locked safely in the metal bonds in the teeth, but can leak slowly into the body, often causing severe illness.

- Some countries, like Sweden, Canada and Germany have either banned or imposed serious limitations on amalgam usage.

<http://www.niddk.nih.gov/Harmful/Harmeff.html>
Harmful Effects of Medicines on the Adult Digestive System
The National Institute of Diabetes and Digestive and Kidney Diseases at the National Institutes of Health
    Written for the patient or layperson.

<http://cpmcnet.columbia.edu/dept/gi/disliv.html>
Diseases of the Liver ★
Howard J. Worman, M.D., Columbia University
    Alphabetical list with hyperlinks to many liver-related disease articles.

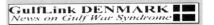

Diseases of the Liver

<http://musom.marshall.edu/chh/DrugInfo/Review/Drug-sun.htm>
Drug-Induced Photosensitivity
Marshall University School of Medicine
    An alphabetical listing of drugs that can cause photosenstivity reactions.

<http://www.nemsn.org/>
National Eosinophilia-Myalgia Syndrome Network
Dumfries, Virginia
    Formed by EMS survivors who ingested contaminated L-tryptophan supplements.

<http://pharminfo.com/pubs/msb/gfj_effect.html>
The Grapefruit Juice Effect
PharmInfo
    Listing of drugs that may be potentiated by being taken with grapefruit juice.

<http://users.cybercity.dk/~ccc11401/home.html>
The Danish Gulf War Veterans Info Team ★
Fanoe, Denmark
    - Information on and links to Gulf War resources.
    - Independent of any official or political influence.

GulfLink DENMARK
News on Gulf War Syndrome

<http://www.gulfweb.org/>
Gulf War Veteran Resource Pages ★
    - Includes the home pages of the National Gulf War Resource Center Inc., Washington, D.C.; the Persian Gulf Veterans Association, Boone, North Carolina; the UK GulfVets, Peterborough, Cambs, UK; and other member organizations.
    - Information about and links to resources for Gulf War Veterans.

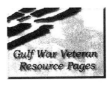

Gulf War Veteran Resource Pages

An award winning site Serving the Gulf War Veteran Community Since 1994

<http://huizen.dds.nl/%7Ehypo/index.htm>
Hypoglycemia Holland Home Page ★★
Lars Idema
- Links to hypoglycemia sites.
- Books and Scientific Literature.
- US and Netherland Organizations.
- Mailing Lists and News Groups.
- Clinical Causes and FAQ's.

CDC Childhood Lead Poisoning Prevention Program

<http://www.cdc.gov/nceh/programs/lead/lead.htm>
CDC Childhood Lead Poisoning Prevention Program ★
Centers for Disease Control, Atlanta, Georgia
- What Every Parent Should Know about Lead Poisoning in Children
- Grants for State- and Community-Based Programs
- Research Publications
- Prevention Workshops
- Screening Guidelines
- Printed copies of the guidance document are available at (888) 232-6789

<http://www.knowlead.com/>
Lead Poison Information
Carolina Environment, Inc., Charlotte, North Carolina
This company markets Know Lead, a test kit available to the general public.

<http://www.nsc.org/ehc/lead.htm>
National Lead Information Center, a division of the National Safety Council H
Washington, D.C.
- Information on lead toxicity.
- Links to other related topics.
- Information available in Spanish

<http://vhp.nus.sg/PID/eng-chi/PID.big5.html>
Poisons Information Database ★★
National University of Singapore
- Listing of natural toxins and poisons.
- Directory of antivenoms around the world.
- Directory of toxicologists around the world.
- Directory of poison control centers around the world.

<http://www.pitt.edu/~martint/pages/poisres.htm>
Poison Information Resources ★★
University of Pittsburgh, Pennsylvania
Links to multiple sources worldwide in various languages.

<http://www.peg.apc.org/%7Enexus/Aspartame.html>
The Bitter Truth about Artificial Sweeteners
Mark Gold, Cambridge, Massachusetts
> Aspartame accounts for over 75 percent of the adverse reactions reported to the U.S. Food and Drug Administration (FDA).

<http://www.digitalnation.com/mshomon/thyroid/>
Thyroid Disease Information Source ★
Mary Shomon, The Mining Company
> Information, articles, and hyperlinks to all aspects of thyroid diseases.

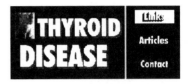

D. *Cutting Edge, Alternative, or Nontradi- tional Medicinal Modalities or Treatments for Emotional Conditions*

> Web sites listed below represent traditional and nontraditional forms of therapy. Their listing does not necessarily constitute an endorsement of their practices or methods.

i. GENERAL RESOURCES

<http://www.pitt.edu/~cbw/altm.html>
The Alternative Medicine Home Page ★★
Falk Library of the Health Sciences, University of Pittsburgh
- Resources on a wide variety of alternative therapeutic techniques are listed alphabetically.
- Many of the listed sites are reviewed.

<http://altmed.od.nih.gov/>
Office of Alternative Medicine
National Institutes of Health, Washington, D.C.

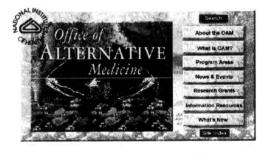

- OAM classifies alternative therapies into the following categories:
  Alternative systems of medical practice (Oriental Medicine, Native American Practices, etc.),
  Bioelectromagnetic Applications (Light Therapy, Electroacupuncture, etc.),
  Diet, Nutrition, Lifestyle Changes (Gerson Therapy, Nutritional Supplements)
  Herbal Medicine,
  Manual Healing (Acupressure, Rolfing, Massage, etc.),
  Mind/Body Control (Music Therapy, Biofeedback),
  Pharmacological and Biological Treatments.
- Fields of Practice has an overview of these six categories.
- Alternative Medicine Research can be accessed using Medline (which has 23 main headings).

<http://www.teleport.com/~mattlmt/>
The Internet International Directory of Alternative/Complementary Medicine Practitioners
The ALTMED Home Page ★★
- This is a free service for providers worldwide to list their services; subscribers can list up to four disciplines of their choosing.
- Consumers can search by continent, country, and local area.

<http://www.dungeon.com/home/cam/rmmc.html>
Complementary Medicine ★★
Research Council for Complementary Medicine, London, UK
- With over 30,000 records, perhaps the most comprehensive database of published complementary medicine research worldwide.
- Sourced from the British Library and Medline databases.
- For requests from health professionals and researchers and not the general public.
- Fee-based service.

<http://www.forthrt.com/~chronicl/archiv.htm#5>
Complementary Medicine Resources ★★
Table of contents includes:
General Reference
Specific Physical/Body Focused Medicine
Specific Mind/Spirit Focused Medicine
General Indices-Pointers
E-Zines, Journals, and Newsletters
Newsgroups
Organizations
Related Links
Networks
Mailing Lists

<http://www.teleport.com/~ibis/ibis.html>
Diverse Medical Information, IBIS: The Interactive Medical Database ★★
Integrative Medical Arts Group, Inc., Beaverton, Oregon
- Reference of 282 common medical conditions with related treatment information from 12 systems of natural medicine and alternative therapies.
- IBIS is a software system for sale to practitioners.

<http://www.hriptc.org/>
Health Research Institute
Naperville, Illinois
HRI is a leading force in the research and treatment of biochemical imbalances.

<http://www.geocities.com/HotSprings/5940/>
The Holistic Health Page ★★
Links to sites worldwide in English, German, and Italian.

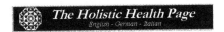

<http://www.europa.com/~itm/>
ITM Online: Chinese, Tibetan, Ayurvedic, Native American, and Thai Medicine ★★
- The Institute for Traditional Medicine, Portland, Oregon, a not-for-profit organization
- Information for patients as well as advanced practitioners.

ii. SPECIFIC MODALITIES OR TREATMENTS

a. Aromatherapy

<http://users.vnet.net/shae/altheal/aroma.html>
Aromatherapy ★
General articles and links to aromatherapy pages.

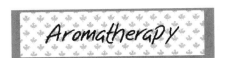

<http://users.ica.net/cnsa/>
Aromatherapy Education: Canadian National School of Aromatherapy
Mississauga, Ontario
Aromatherapy oils and information about certification.

<http://leydet.com/air/>
A.I.R. Aromatherapy Institute and Research
Fair Oaks, California
Aromatherapy certification courses and seminars.

<http://www.imm.org.pl/bird/list.htm>
Bird's Encyclopedia of Aromatherapy ★
Index of oils and their properties.

<http://www.eskimo.com/~hhnews/naha/>
National Association for Holistic Aromatherapy
Boulder, Colorado
Resource clearinghouse for ideas and information about AT.

b. Ayurvedic Medicine

<http://www.healthy.net/library/articles/ayurvedic/ayurintro.htm>
Ayurvedic Medicine: A Brief Introduction and Guide
Dr. Vasant Lad, The Ayurvedic Institute

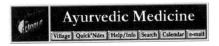

Ayurveda places great emphasis on prevention and encourages maintaining health by paying close attention to balance in one's life through right thinking, diet, lifestyle, and herbs.

<http://www.niam.com/index1.html>
The National Institute of Ayurvedic Medicine
Brewster, New York
> People should not try to medicate themselves or others with any of the plants referred to here without the guidance of an individual fully trained in Ayurveda.

c. Botanical, Herbal, and Horticultural Therapies

<http://www.skynet.co.uk/bach/>
Bach Flower Remedies
- Dr. Edward Bach (pronounced BATCH) developed a system of 38 flower remedies that can address emotional conditions.
- These remedies, which can be used alongside conventional medications, are not a substitute for medical treatment.

<http://chili.rt66.com/hrbmoore/HOMEPAGE/HomePage.html>
Southwest School of Botanical Medicine ★
Bisbee, Arizona
> Medicinal plant images, information on and links to botanical medicine sites.

<http://www.treasureofeast.com/>
Concentrated Chinese Herbs ★
Blue Light Inc.
> This site includes:
> An Introduction to Chinese Medicine
> The Benefits of Concentrated Herbs
> Common Ailments and Recommended Patent Herbs
> Herbal Catalog

Henriette's Herbal Homepage

<http://sunsite.unc.edu/herbmed/>
Henriette's Herbal Home Page ★
Henriette Kress, Helsinki, Finland
> Herbal FAQ's, archives, plant pictures, links to medicinal plant sites.

<http://www.medherb.com/>
Medical Herbalism: A Clinical Newsletter for the Herbal Practitioner
Bergner Communications, Boulder, Colorado
- To strengthen the herbal practitioner, to preserve and develop the science and art of herbal medicine, and to promote communication and sharing of clinical methods and experiences.
- This newsletter is available by subscription only.

Welcome to the Herb Society (UK) Home Page

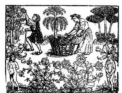

<http://sunsite.unc.edu/herbmed/HerbSociety/>
UK Herb Society Home Page ★
- A variety of information about herbs and their usefulness.
- Links to herbal sites.

<http://www.nnlm.nlm.nih.gov/pnr/uwmhg/>
The University of Washington Medicinal Herb Garden ★
Seattle, Washington
> A resource for herbalists, medics, and botanists of all levels. Not a source of medical advice or a guide to self-medication.

<http://http.tamu.edu:8000/~pnw3384/ahta.html>
American Horticultural Therapy Association
Gaithersburg, Maryland
> Horticultural therapy is a process utilizing plants and horticultural activities to improve the social, educational, psychological and physical adjustment of persons thus improving their body, mind and spirits.

American Horticultural
Therapy Association

<http://aggie-horticulture.tamu.edu/horther/index.html>
Horticultural Therapy ★
> Information about and links to people/plant therapeutics.

d. Chiropractic

<http://pages.prodigy.com/CT/doc/doc.html>
Chiro-Web ★★
> Links and information on chiropractic around the world.

e. Homeopathy

<http://www.dungeon.com/~cam/index.html>
Homeopathy Home Page ★★
> A worldwide homeopathic Internet resources list.

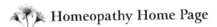

Homeopathy Home Page

<http://www.ihr.com/homeopat/research.html>
Scientific Evidence for Homeopathic Medicine ★
Dana Ullman, M.P.H., Berkeley, California
> Excerpted from *The Consumer's Guide to Homeopathy*

f. Naturopathic Medicine

http/www.pandamedicine.com/>
Naturopathic Medicine Network ★
Pandamedicine Natural Pharmacy
> A keyword search for topics related to N.M. is available.

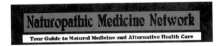

g. Osteopathic Medicine

<http://www.rscom.com/osteo/>
Osteopathic Medicine: International WWW Resource Website
Rosegarth Communications Ltd., Mansfield, NOTTS, UK
> A growing site with info on OM.

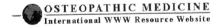

h. Individual Nontraditional Medications

<http://www.coldeeze-net.com/>
The Official Cold-Eeze Site
The Quig Corporation
> Information on the first product that cures (or at least shortens) the common cold.

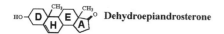 Dehydroepiandrosterone

<http://www.naples.net/~nfn03605/>
DHEA Home Page
J.M. Howard
> All-purpose information site for dehydroepiandrosterone.

<http://www.natrol.com/products/dhea-wp.html>
DHEA White Paper
Natrol, Inc.
> Legal status, product efficacy, and general information about DHEA.

<http://www.ginseng.ca/gi02007.htm>
Scientific Studies on the Effects of Ginseng ★
Herbal Direct Ginseng Products
> Many scientific experiments have been done on the effects of ginseng.

<http://www.ginkoba.org/ginkben.htm>
Ginkoba Benefits ★
Boehringer Ingelheim Pharmaceuticals
> Information about Ginkoba, its benefits, and studies showing its effectiveness.

<http://www.usdoctor.com/gh.htm>
Growth Hormone: The First Anti-Aging Medication?
Edward M. Lichten, M.D., P.C.
> Dr. Lichten is a proponent of the benefits of hGH for adults.

<http://www.uhc.com/resource/rhghbody.html>
Recombinant Human Growth Hormone
> A more scientific approach examining indications for hGH and diagnostic criteria for its administration.

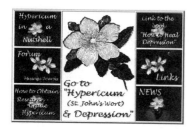

<http://www.hypericum.com/>
The Hypericum (St. John's Wort) and Depression Home Page
Peter McWilliams, Harold H. Bloomfield, M.D.
> The on-line version of the printed book *Hypericum and Depression* is available without charge.

<http://www.melatonin.com/eads.htm>
Melatonin Central
Worldwide Labs
>   General FAQ and Medical FAQ sections.

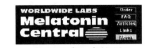

<http://home.comm.net/~healthylink/>
Pycnogenol
Health Link
>   Includes general information and clinical monographs for general use and for ADD.

<http://www.ceri.com/>
Smart Drug News: The Newsletter of Cognitive Enhancement and Longevity ★
Cognitive Enhancement Research Institute, Menlo Park, California
>   • FAQ's about smart drugs and nutrients.
>   • Smart drug updates.
>   • Importing and buying smart drugs.

<http://www.healthlink.com.au/nat_lib/htm-data/htm-supp/supps7.htm>
L-Tryptophan
HealthLink Natural Resources
>   General information about indications and precautions.

E. *Food and Nutrition*

<http://allergy.pair.com/additives/foodad.htm>
Food Additives ★
Northern Allergy Center, Byron Bay, Australia
>   What you always wanted to know about food additives but had no one to ask.

<http://www.nidlink.com/~mastent/>
Mastering Food Allergies ★
Mast Enterprises, Inc., Coeur d'Alene, Idaho
>   • All-purpose information about the most common food allergies.
>   • Allergen-free recipes.

<http://arborcom.com/>
Arbor Nutrition Guide ★★
Dr. Tony Helman
>   • Information for family physicians, dietitians, patients, hospitals, universities.
>   • Some resources are available in Spanish and German.

<http://members.aol.com/nutrigenie/index.html>
NutriGenie
NutriGenie Publishers
> A variety of software programs to help with diet, nutrition, and weight control.

<http://virtualjax.com/sprayit/index.html>
Spray Vitamins
Vitamist
> A variety of different vitamin combinations in spray formula.

<http://www.mineraltoddy.com/>
Colloidal Minerals Liquid Vitamins
The Toddy Shop
> Liquid vitamin products and research studies and articles on nutrition and colloidal

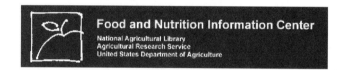

<http://www.nal.usda.gov/fnic/>
Food and Nutrition Information Center ★★
United States Department of Agriculture
> • This site includes:
> Publications and databases
> Foodborne Illness Education Information Center
> Healthy School Meals Resource System
> Index of Food and Nutrition Internet Resources
> Diet information produced by other USDA agencies
> • A keyword search is available.

<http://www.vegsoc.org/>
Health and Nutrition ★★
> • General information on nutrition and physical and emotional diseases and disorders.
> • From the UK Vegetarian Society.

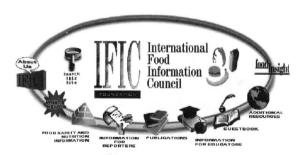

<http://ificinfo.health.org/>
International Food Information Council
Washington, D.C.
> • Formed in 1985, IFIC offers programs and activities sponsored by a number of leading food and beverage companies.
> • To serve as the critical link between the scientific community, food manufacturers, health professionals, government officials and the news media.

<http://www.monash.edu.au/IUNS/>
International Union of Nutritional Sciences ★★
Monash University, Australia
> This site contains:
>> Links to other international organizations
>> Food and nutrition information
>> Nutrition education
>> Nutrition events
>> Nutrition atlas, an international directory of food and nutrition sources

<http://www.ag.uiuc.edu/~food-lab/nat/>
Nutrition Analysis Tool v.1.1
University of Illinois—Urbana/Champaign
- A web-based program that analyzes foods for different nutrients.
- Free and easy to use.
- Analysis can be saved to hard drive or disk.

<http://www.ahsc.arizona.edu/nutrition/>
Nutrition and Health ★★
Arizona Health Services Library, University of Arizona, Tucson
> The site contains links to and information on:
>> Diseases and Health
>> Nutrition and Foods Industry
>> Grants and Research
>> Exercise and Fitness
>> Nutrition WWW
>> Consumer Information
>> Foods and Recipes
>> Foods and Nutrients
>> Herbs and Herbal Medicine
>> International Nutrition Sites
>> Food Safety
>> Electronic Forums
>> Vitamins and Antioxidants
>> Libraries and Universities
>> Dietetics Sources
>> Clinical Nutrition

<http://www.thorne.com/townsend/nov/null.html>
Nutrition and Mental Illness: Sampling of the Current Scientific Literature ★★
> Listing of articles discussing nutrition and various disorders.

F. *Associations, Companies, Miscellaneous Web Sites, Products, Medical Categorizations*

\<http://www.ecnp.nl/specials/welcome.htm\>
European College of Neuropsychopharmacology
The Netherlands
- Established in 1986 to encourage research and facilitate communication of ideas in the convergent disciplines.
- ECNP has established:
  fellowships for young scientists
  research awards
  a scientific journal, *European Neuropsychopharmacology*

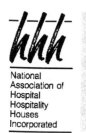

National Association of Hospital Hospitality Houses Incorporated

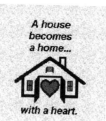

A house becomes a home... *with a heart.*

\<http://visit-usa.com/hhh/\>
National Association of Hospital Hospitality Houses Incorporated
Bethesda, Maryland
- A membership organization of hospital hospitality (Ronald McDonald-style) programs.
- Members are listed by state.

\<http://WWW.NPATH.ORG/\>
National Patient Air Transport Helpline
The Air Care Alliance, Virginia Beach, Virginia
Free information and referral for those who need to move a loved one to distant locations after an illness or accident, health care professionals needing to find cost-effective ways to move patients and their family members, and volunteer pilots who wish to serve with the AirCare Alliance.

\<http://www.alza.com/\>
The ALZA Corporation
Palo Alto, California
Development and commercialization of pharmaceutical products using advanced drug delivery technologies, including osmotic systems.

\<http://www.ramex.com/\>
RAmEx: Rampertab American Exports Inc.
Los Angeles, California
- An international distributor of multimedia titles for medical professionals.
- Includes medical books, videos, slides, and CD ROM, medical audio tapes and software.

<http://www.medicom.com>
The Internet Medical Products Guide
Medical Internet Communications, Inc.
> A service providing information on the latest products and services.

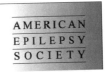

Welcome to
The Internet Medical Products Guide
The Electronic Index of Medical Products and Services.

<http://www.pemed.com/intro.htm>
Used Medical Equipment
PEMED, Denver, Colorado
> 25,000 square feet of used medical equipment at 20 to 40 percent of retail price.

G. *Epilepsy Information*

<http://www.aesnet.org/>
American Epilepsy Society ★
Hartford, Connecticut
> Seeks to promote interdisciplinary communication, scientific investigation, and exchange of clinical information about epilepsy.

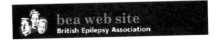

<http://www.epilepsy.org.uk/>
British Epilepsy Association ★
Site sponsored by Glaxo-Wellcome
> A membership organization with branches throughout the UK.

<http://www.epinet.org.au>
EpiNet: Epilepsy Association of Victoria, Australia
Information Kits
> Information on the rights of people with epilepsy

<http://www.epilepsy.ca/>
Epilepsy Canada
Montreal, Quebec
> Not-for-profit organization to promote and support research into all aspects of epilepsy and to create awareness and understanding about epilepsy through educational programs.

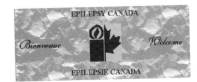

<http://www.bgsm.edu/bgsm/surg-sci/ns/epilepsy.html>
Epilepsy Index ★★
- Department of Neurosurgery, Bowman Gray School of Medicine, Wake Forest University
- Information and referral to 8,000 callers a year at (800) 642-0500.
- List of organizations providing support and education about epilepsy.
- Many other links.

<http://www.squish.com/rickloek/ketopages/>
Ketogenic Diet ★
Rick Loek
- Information and links.
- Not intended to be a source of medical advice.

<http://www-leland.stanford.edu/group/ketodiet/>
Ketogenic Diet ★
Packard Children's Hospital, Stanford University Medical Center
- Resources for parents.
- Keto-Diet mailing list.
- Pediatric Neurology
- Diet Meal Planner Worksheet section.
- FAQ's

<http://www.mynchen.demon.co.uk/>
Ketogenic Resource ★
- Information on the ketogenic diet and related matters like epilepsy and cerebral palsy in young children.
- Not a source of medical advice.

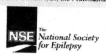

<http://bay.erg.ion.bpmf.ac.uk/NSEhome/>
National Society for Epilepsy, UK ★
Gerrards Cross, Buckinghamshire, UK
  Information applies to the UK; legal regulations relating to employment and driving and the names of anti-epileptic drugs will differ from country to country.

<http://starbase.neosoft.com/~cara/epilepsy.html>
Epilepsy Resources ★★
Sarah Pleasant and Terri Stimmel
- 100 books on epilepsy in the Bookstore section.
- Two IRC chat channels for epilepsy.
- Many other links.

<http://canddwilson.com/tbi/tbiepil.htm>
Traumatic Brain Injury and Epilepsy Page ★
- Information on TBI and ABI
- Epilepsy mailing lists.
- Service dog information.
- Litigation information.
- Survivor's WWW home pages.

H. *Mailing Lists*

Alternative Medical Forum News on
    American OnLine
listserv@listserv.aol.com
SUBSCRIBE AHHPULSE

Traumatic Brain Injury Professionals
listserv@maelstrom.stjohns.edu
SUBSCRIBE TBI-PROF

Brain Tumor Research/Support
listserv@mitvma.mit.edu
SUBSCRIBE BRAINTMR

Comparative Medicine List
listserv@wuvmd.wustl.edu
SUBSCRIBE COMPMED

Herbarium Intermountain and
    Pacific Northwest Discussion
listserv@idbsu.idbsu.edu
SUBSCRIBE HERB-L

Homeopathy, Flower Remedies and
    Flower Essence Forum
listserv@listserv.aol.com
SUBSCRIBE HOMEOPATHY

Medical Marijuana
listproc@ns2.calyx.net
SUBSCRIBE MEDMJ

Medical Journal Discussion Club
listserv@brownvm.brown.edu
SUBSCRIBE JMEDCLUB

Medical Libraries Discussion Listserv
listserv@listserv.acsu.buffalo.edu
SUBSCRIBE MEDLIB-L

Pharmacology
mailbase@mailbase.ac.uk
JOIN PHARMACOLOGY-TLTP

Pharmacology
mailbase@mailbase.ac.uk
JOIN PHARMACOLOGY-COMMS

Child Pharmacology
listserv@maelstrom.stjohns.edu
SUBSCRIBE CAPHARM Your Name

Pharmacology Seminar
listserv@lsumc.edu
SUBSCRIBE PHARM-SEMINAR

Psychopharmacology
majordomo@psycom.net
SUB PSYCHO-PHARM

Medicinal and Aromatic Plants Discussion
listserv@vm3090.ege.edu.tr
SUBSCRIBE HERB

Prozac Discussion
listserv@maelstrom.stjohns.edu
SUBSCRIBE PROZAC

Psychology/Psychiatry Outcome Research in
    Psychopharmacology
listserv@maelstrom.stjohns.edu
SUBSCRIBE PSY-PHAR

Medical Resource Development
listserv@maelstrom.stjohns.edu
SUBSCRIBE MMATRIX-L

Medical Students
listserv@listserv.indiana.edu
SUB MED-STUDENTS-L Your Name

Palliative Medicine
mailbase@mailbase.ac.uk
JOIN PALLIATIVE-MEDICINE

Thyroid Discussion
listserv@maelstrom.stjohns.edu
SUBSCRIBE THYROID

Toxicology
listserv@syrres.com
SUB ToxList Your Name